David O. Moberg, PhD
Editor

Aging and Spirituality
Spiritual Dimensions of Aging Theory, Research, Practice, and Policy

Pre-publication
REVIEWS,
COMMENTARIES,
EVALUATIONS . . .

More pre-publication
REVIEWS, COMMENTARIES, EVALUATIONS . . .

"The focus of this edited book is the special significance of spirituality in later life, but the authors do an admirable job of applying a life-course framework. One argument for the significance of spirituality in later life is found in Moberg's consideration of spirituality in social gerontological theories. This chapter provides a blueprint for studying the ways in which spirituality and aging interact in social life. Indeed, for social scientists, perhaps the most important question raised in this book is whether spirituality is outside the domain of scientific research. The book does a wonderful job of identifying a myriad of scientifically researchable questions on a host of topics ranging from the spiritual role of elders in social life to whether spirituality and religiosity increase with age. The book is particularly rich in practical applications: How does spirituality shape primary health care, hospice care, social work, or counseling with older adults? It will be an invaluable resource for professionals engaged in delivering services to older people whether in sectarian or secular institutions. Indexes and suggested readings also make the book very convenient to use. Moberg has provided both the scholarly and professional communities with a timely resource for those interested in aging and spirituality."

Kenneth F. Ferraro
Professor of Sociology and Director,
Gerontology Program,
Purdue University,
Lafayette, IN

"Dr. David O. Moberg, an outstanding sociologist in the field of aging, has edited this survey and introduction to spirituality in social gerontology. It is an important tool for integrating the central theme of old age into the practice, care, and research of the helping professions, including health care professionals, social workers, counselors, chaplains, nursing coordinators and homes, and those associated with mental health institutions and churches.

Dr. Moberg, in one of his several excellent chapters, stresses the importance of elder's spiritual life reviews or spiritual autobiographies, for the current generation and for the elder.

I recommend this book to all health professionals, well-informed el-ders and denomination leaders, and politicians. With the massive increase in elders soon expected in the American population, the huge resource potentially represented by this group, as respected teachers of wisdom, cher- ishers of the cultural story and values, counselors of the young, and enablers of courageous concern in the community, is far too important to our country's future not to recognize it politically and encourage it in every aspect of our culture."

Elisabeth McSherry, MD, MPH
National VHA DSS Deputy Director
of Data Systems Development,
Adjunct Associate Professor,
Department of Community
and Family Health,
Dartmouth Medical School

Aging and Spirituality
Spiritual Dimensions of Aging Theory, Research, Practice, and Policy

THE HAWORTH PASTORAL PRESS
Rev. James W. Ellor, DMin, DCSW, CGP
Melvin A. Kimble, PhD
Co-Editors in Chief

Aging and Spirituality
Spiritual Dimensions of Aging Theory, Research, Practice, and Policy

David O. Moberg, PhD
Editor

The Haworth Pastoral Press®
An Imprint of The Haworth Press, Inc.
New York • London • Oxford

Published by

The Haworth Pastoral Press ®, an imprint of The Haworth Press, Inc., 10 Alice Street, Binghamton, NY 13904-1580

Scripture quotations taken from *The Holy Bible,* New International Version. Copyright 1973, 1978, 1984 by International Bible Society.

Cover design by Jennifer M. Gaska.

Library of Congress Cataloging-in-Publication

Aging and spirituality : spiritual dimensions of aging theory, research, practice, and policy / David O. Moberg, editor.
     p. cm.
   Includes bibliographical references (p.) and indexes.
   ISBN 0-7890-0938-2 (hard : alk. paper)—ISBN 0-7890-0939-0 (soft : alk. paper)
   1. Spirituality. 2. Aged—Religious life. 3. Aging—Religious aspects. I. Moberg, David O.

BL625.4 .A35 2001
291.4'084'6—dc21   00-057516

CONTENTS

ABOUT THE EDITOR

David O. Moberg, PhD, is Sociology Professor Emeritus at Marquette University, where he has taught a broad range of courses, including sociology of religion, social gerontology, and religion and aging. He has been co-editor of the annual series *Research in the Social Scientific Study of Religion* since its founding in 1989, and he is the author of more than 200 professional articles and a dozen books, including *The Church and the Older Person* (with Robert M. Gray) and the edited volume *Spiritual Well-Being: Sociological Perspective*s. He is a former editor of the *Review of Religious Research* and the *Journal of the American Scientific Affiliation,* and he continues to serve on the boards of several professional journals.

CONTRIBUTORS

Edith Anne Glascock Angeli is a volunteer in the Milwaukee Hospice Homecare and Residence and a coordinator of food drives for a food pantry. Her BA in business management with support in professional communications was earned at Alverno College, and her MA in public service with specialization in health care administration is from Marquette University.

Joanne Armatowski, SSND, is a School Sister of Notre Dame in the Milwaukee Province currently employed as the Director of Pastoral Care at St. Joseph Convent, Campbellsport, Wisconsin. Her education includes an MA in public service with a specialization in health care administration from Marquette University and an MA as a reading specialist and elementary school administrator. She has taught elementary and junior high school students and served as a school administrator. During ten years as an administrative leader in her religious community, she has worked with its elderly members and served on its task force to renovate its skilled care facility into an assisted and well-elderly facility. She is a member of the St. Joan Antida High School Foundation Board in Milwaukee and of the St. Francis Home Board in Fond du Lac, Wisconsin.

Robert J. Best, NHA, is the Director of Wildwood Highlands Senior Apartments, Menomonee Falls, Wisconsin. A licensed health care administrator, he has twenty years of experience working with older adults in retirement communities, assisted living facilities, nursing homes, and community settings. His BS with a major in psychology is from Carroll College and his MA in public service with specialization in gerontology is from Marquette University. He is also a fellow in the Wisconsin Geriatric Education Center and vice president of the Waukesha Interfaith Caregiving Network. He is the co-author of *I'll Never Forget Our Home* (Montgomery Media, 1991), a guidebook for older adults, and *Memories of a Home* (Paulist Press, 1993).

He has presented papers at the American Society on Aging, National Council on Aging, National Reminiscence Conference, Coalition of Wisconsin Aging Groups, American Medical Directors, and other conventions.

Ann Driscoll-Lamberg has been a hospital-link case manager in the Community Options Program of Waukesha (WI) County Human Services for eight years. In previous counseling employment, she was a discharge planner at St. Luke's Hospital in Racine, Wisconsin, and a benefit specialist with older adults at St. Joseph's Hospital in Milwaukee. Her BSW is from Mount Mary College and her MA in public service with specialization in gerontology is from Marquette University.

Nils Friberg is Professor of Pastoral Care at Bethel Theological Seminary, St. Paul, Minnesota, from which he earned his BD degree. His PhD dissertation at the University of Iowa was on assessment of the religious coping of women cancer patients. He is a licensed marriage and family therapist with broad experience in counseling, parish consultation, and hospital and police chaplaincies that often require attending to the deaths of elderly persons and ministering to bereaved spouses and family members. Other experience includes public relations, pastorates, parish consultation services, and nine years as a missionary in Brazil. In his teaching he has processed thousands of seminarians' verbatim accounts of pastoral care and counseling encounters, most of which were with elderly people. He is a member of the Midwest regional standards committee of the Association for Clinical Pastoral Education and co-author of the award-winning *Before the Fall: Prevention of Pastoral Sexual Misconduct* (Liturgical Press, 1998).

Carol A. Nickasch is a dental hygiene instructor at Milwaukee Area Technical College and a dental hygienist at the Milwaukee Protestant Home. Her BA in dental hygiene is from Marquette University, her MS in adult education is from the University of Wisconsin-Milwaukee, and her MA in public service with specialization in gerontology is from Marquette University. She has been a Professed Secular Franciscan for sixteen years, during which she has served the Secular Franciscan Order as vice minister of the La Verna region (Wisconsin and Upper Michigan) and held local offices in the St. Francis and Clare Fraternity. She is a Geriatrics Fellow in the Wisconsin Geriatric Education Center.

Pamela Lynn Schultz-Hipp is vice president of ChiroTechAmerica, Inc., a national chiropractic administrative service company for health maintenance organizations and preferred provider organizations. Her BA degree with a major in communications is from the University of Wisconsin-Whitewater, and her MA in public service with specialization in health care administration is from Marquette University. She is co-author of *Managed Care and Chiropractic Rehabilitation: A Continuum* (American Chiropractic Rehabilitation Board, 2000), and she serves as a consultant for independent physicians and health care organizations.

Allison E. Soerens is a Geriatric Nurse Practitioner in Aurora Health Care, Sheboygan, Wisconsin. She earned her BS degree in nursing at the University of Wisconsin-Eau Claire and her MS in geriatric nursing from Marquette University. She was the recipient of the 1997 Marquette Gerontology Nursing Scholarship for academic excellence. Allison is certified as a Geriatric Nurse Practitioner by the American Nurses Credentialing Center, and as an Advance Practice Nurse Prescriber by the State of Wisconsin Department of Regulation and Licensing.

Stephanie Sue Stein was appointed director of the Milwaukee County Department on Aging in 1993 following a distinguished career as senior director of older adult programs in the Social Development Commission. She earned her BA from the University of Wisconsin-Milwaukee and is completing her MA in Public Service with specialization in gerontology at Marquette University. She teaches public policy in aging programs at Marquette University and is a guest lecturer at the University of Wisconsin-Milwaukee and Concordia University Wisconsin. She writes a quarterly column for *AGEnda,* her department's newsletter, and writes, speaks, and lectures locally and nationally on aging issues. She was a delegate at the 1995 White House Conference on Aging, and in 1999 she received the Service to Seniors award of the National Committee to Preserve Social Security and Medicare.

Derrel R. Watkins is Oubri A. Poppele Chair Professor of Health and Welfare Ministries at Saint Paul School of Theology, Kansas City, Missouri, and a professor of social work emeritus at Southwestern Baptist Theological Seminary. His MSW degree with emphasis in gerontology is from the University of Georgia, and his PhD is from Southwestern Baptist Theological Seminary with a dissertation on the relationship of the action principle to prognosis in group psycho-therapy. He also completed postdoctoral studies in human service administration at the University of Texas at Arlington and has been a researcher for the National Interfaith Coalition on Aging. He has presented papers at meetings of many professional associations and contributed articles to various journals and books on social work practice. His latest book is *Christian Social Ministry: An Introduction* (Broadman and Holman, 1994).

Foreword

The Pastoral Press book program has been developed to offer helping professionals useful books that address topics that (1) bridge science and theology, (2) offer wholistic approaches to ministry, and (3) contain practical insights that assist professionals and volunteers who work with older adults. This series offers timely, cutting edge manuscripts that will enhance any library with insights for practice. The texts are written by authors who have demonstrated their skill in social science and ministry.

Each text addresses topics that are written from an interfaith position. From this perspective the faith position of the author is affirmed, yet not offered as exclusive, allowing the reader to affirm his or her own faith in light of the topic being explored. It is our hope that this text will offer the reader insights and techniques to enhance his or her own work.

Editors of this program are affiliated with the Center for Aging, Religion, and Spirituality (CARS). CARS offers numerous interfaith programs for professionals working with older adults. These programs are housed at Luther Seminary in St. Paul, Minnesota. More information about CARS can be found at <www.Luthersem.edu/cars>.

Aging and Spirituality offers insights into theory, data, and practice that can be applied to the needs of older adults. The book also provides an administrative and public policy approach. Edited by a key member of the religious and aging community, David Moberg offers fresh reflection on each topic as well as his vision of the continuing challenges of this field. This important book will be helpful for persons working in research as well as in direct practice with older adults.

Reverend James W. Ellor, PhD, DMin, DCSW, CGP
Editor in Chief
The Haworth Pastoral Press

Acknowledgments

Hundreds of people have contributed directly or indirectly to the making of this book. Much of our indebtedness to others is evident from the abundant references to work that others have done. It is impossible to list all of the spouses and other family members, colleagues, librarians, employers, friends, and even strangers upon whom we have called for inspiration, manuscript reviews, secretarial and office services, bits of information, or other support to us as editor and authors. The chapter authors have been very cooperative even when I, as editor, returned early drafts for revisions or asked for clarification of details that I felt would help you who are the readers. To all of them, and especially to series editor James Ellor and the Haworth staff, we extend our sincere thanks.

David O. Moberg

Introduction

During the closing years of the twentieth century, the recognition that spirituality is a very important contributor to the total well-being of older adults expanded rapidly. Scientific research, clinical observations, and the humanistic scholarship that explored connections between the religiousness and spirituality of people, on the one hand, and aspects of their whole-person wellness, on the other, increased the evidence that spiritual health is strongly and positively related to their overall well-being. This strengthened the conviction that human services of all kinds must include attention to the spiritual nature and needs of people.

Evidence and awareness of the importance of spirituality to wellness in almost every domain of life, if not indeed in all, have increased the need of people in geriatrics, health and medicine, social work, the ministry, counseling, and all the other human service professions for resources to help guide their activities related to spiritual needs. The numbers and proportion of the population who are elderly are steadily increasing. Almost all contemporary adults in due time attain the status of senior citizens, the age group that is the most aware of spiritual concerns. Spirituality infuses human existence and influences every area of human activity, so studying it is personally relevant and helpful for everyone at all ages.

This book confirms the pervasiveness of human spirituality, suggests how it can be integrated into the theoretical framework of social gerontology, summarizes research on its importance in the lives of senior adults, illustrates ways to enhance spiritual wellness through various human service professions and by actions of older persons themselves, and points to both pertinent accomplishments and problematic contexts of relevant professions and public policy. It reveals significant ways to improve spiritual health, shows the importance of

assessing spiritual needs, illustrates how laypersons and professionals contribute to improving the spiritual wellness of individuals, offers basic principles for research on spirituality, and gives practical
guidelines for evaluating how best to do such research and assessments.

Although it is logically organized into four interrelated parts,
each chapter can be read as a unit and in any order that appeals to the
reader.

QUESTIONS ANSWERED

Readers will find answers, some direct and forthright, others indirect and implicit, to many questions in the following pages. Among
them are the following examples:

- Is spirituality the same as religion, or are they related in some other
  way?
- Is spirituality outside the domain of scientific research?
- What are the spiritual needs of typical people in late life?
- Is there any solid evidence that prayer changes things?
- How is spirituality related to physical and mental health?
- Does spirituality matter when people know they are dying?
- How is spiritual care relevant to the helping professions?
- By what methods or techniques can we evaluate or measure spiri-
  tual wellness and assess the outcomes of activities intended to en-
  hance it?

The answers to those and many other questions are tucked away in
the chapters of this book. The first three chapters summarize conceptual and theoretical foundations for understanding and applying spirituality. They are followed by three that summarize the growing body
of research on the subject and provide guidelines for doing research
and evaluating research projects.

The third section consists of professional and practical applications in health care settings, hospices, counseling, social work, personal life, and chaplaincies, especially in long-term care facilities.
These chapters demonstrate many of the ways in which attention to
spiritual care can be incorporated into pastoral work and all of the
helping professions.

The last part addresses public policy issues related to spirituality from the perspective of the need for long-term care that many people experience during old age, provides guidelines for evaluations and research, and summarizes representative practical and scholarly challenges for future development that are related to the spiritual nature of humanity.

Finally, the annotated list of recommended readings shows that this book overlaps with several others, although its scope and approach to the subject are unique, so it does not duplicate any of them. The indexes of names and subjects make it easy to locate related publications and in-depth reports on many topics for further study and specialized reference needs.

WHO SHOULD READ THIS BOOK?

As an introduction to and survey of the entire field of aging and spirituality, this book can serve as a textbook or supplementary reading for persons already in or preparing for careers that serve aging and elderly people. These include teaching and research, geriatrics and gerontology, the health professions, social work, religious studies, theology, the social/behavioral sciences, or other disciplines and occupations. The perspectives, principles, and procedures applied in each human service profession that is discussed are not vocationally limited; they can serve as models or examples to all of the others, including those that are not specifically mentioned.

Alhough this overview of spirituality and aging will be of primary interest to service providers and their students, it also will prove interesting and useful to older persons who are curious about their own experiences with religion and spirituality and how they are similar to or different from those of other people. It will aid those who wish to enhance their own spiritual well-being or who desire to help others spiritually. They may want to know whether spiritual growth is possible without increasing their personal problems in other domains of their lives. Will giving attention to spirituality aggravate or alleviate the losses that tend to pile up during the later years of the life span? Will it intensify deprivation and depression during the aging process, or is it more likely to enhance personal satisfactions and joys?

Professional people who specialize in gerontology and geriatrics will benefit greatly from these overviews of research and clinical practice, all of which acknowledge that spirituality is ontologically real, not just a figment of the human imagination or folklore. So, too, will directors of pastoral care, chaplains, pastors, social workers, health professionals, sociologists, psychologists, theologians, and religious educators, especially when their focus of attention is spirituality, aging, or both.

In effect, therefore, this book can serve as either a primary or a supplemental text for educational programs, workshops, and continuing education training for professional people, and it can be a very helpful resource for discussion circles and educational forums in senior citizen centers and religious groups. All libraries that serve the general public, educational institutions, or specialized agencies related to religion, aging, or spirituality should add it to their collections.

THE AUTHORS

As the Contributors section indicates, all of the authors are superbly qualified to make their respective contributions. They are professional persons actively engaged in administrative positions, education, or professional services related to aging and elderly people. Their training and experience is based upon various fields of study, among them nursing, social work, psychology, sociology, business administration, theology, pastoral care, dental hygiene, and health care administration. Based upon such diverse perspectives, research, professional applications, and experience, their chapters comprise a very useful and rich introduction to both the how-to-do-it and the scholarly aspects of spirituality and aging. They constitute a well-rounded interdisciplinary survey that fills a major gap in current resources.

Those who use this book as a stepping-stone to in-depth knowledge of religious gerontology as a whole or to any of the specific topics included will find more detailed information in the dozens of works mentioned in the recommended readings and chapter references. To my knowledge, no other book covers the same scope and integrative approach to the subject of aging and spirituality.

CONCEPTUAL AND THEORETICAL FOUNDATIONS

These first three chapters provide the basis for attention to spirituality. Why is it an important subject? How is it related to religion? What are some perceptions of its influence on personal lives and professional practice? Is there still a spiritual role for older Americans, or were such roles limited to earlier and preliterate societies?

Then we shall suggest some of the ways in which spirituality has been or could be incorporated into and understood better through the perspectives of theories in the field of social gerontology. Since professional work of every kind, as well as leadership in religious and other organizations, is directed by known or unrecognized theoretical orientations, understanding them lays the groundwork for both academic and applied professional services and activities. They will help to improve the self-understanding of those who serve aging people and provide a firmer foundation for much of their work.

Chapter 1

The Reality and Centrality
of Spirituality

David O. Moberg

An old spiritual says that "Everybody talkin' 'bout heaven ain't a-goin' there." Spirituality is similar. There is much talk about it, but most people are uncertain about its definition, and many are not sure they possess it. In a 1998 Gallup poll, 82 percent of American adults said that they felt a need to experience spiritual growth, but only 13 percent had a deep, transforming faith (Gallup, 1999).

The "spiritual" label has become so pervasive in popular culture that Lentini refers to the electronic "global entertainment village" as "the new worldwide temple of pop polytheism" (1999, p. 20). Many people have a personal implicit religion of experiences, feelings, ultimate commitments, foci of interaction, and intensive concerns for which they live, even if they reject conventional religious faith (see Bailey, 1998; Wuthnow, 1998). Their visible religion is not the same as their invisible spirituality, although religion and spirituality are often treated as if they are identical.

Meanwhile, in professional and academic circles there has been a long series of "ways of the spirit coming and going as movements of the hour. . . . Their passing or still lasting popularity and validity . . . is a powerful testimony to the hunger for transcendent meaning" (Van Kaam, 1992, p. 331).

Although spirituality, along with cognates like spiritual, is a widely used word, precise interpretations of it are rare even in professional circles, and there is no universal definition that can be operationalized and measured (Koenig, 1997, pp. 70-71). It is strongly interwoven with references to traditional religions, although many Americans now are into spirituality while rejecting religion (Cimino and Lattin, 1999). If asked to explain spirituality, most people describe persons or groups they believe to be spiritual or resort to practices or ideologies alleged to promote spirituality. But listing the characteristics of any given phenomenon is not the same as defining it, and the same is true of specifying the means by which it can be attained. Is spirituality real or imaginary?

THE SPIRITUAL NATURE OF HUMANITY

In 1965 between transportation connections from Oxford, England, to my home, I visited Foyle's in London, then billed as "the world's largest bookstore." Among used books under sociology I saw a title, *The True Life,* that seemed misplaced. Curiously, I pulled it off the shelf and discovered a striking subtitle, *The Sociology of the Supernatural.* In it Sturzo (1947), an Italian sociologist, emphasized that "the true life" of humanity exists within the context of the supernatural, whether they realize it or not. The supernatural is not a separate section of social life juxtaposed to the natural as its opposite so that individuals may accept or reject it at will. Instead, the supernatural and natural order meet in people. Even those who deny the supernatural root and branch of the religious life in a search for purely natural explanations of religion are involved, albeit negatively, with a sociology of the supernatural. "In studying society in its complex wholeness, it is found to exist within the atmosphere of the supernatural" (p. 17).

Spirituality is possibly the most significant aspect of that supernatural atmosphere enveloping all earthly and human reality. As we continue to emerge from the rationalistic and positivistic worldview that has dominated Western civilization for a century or more, there is an increasing recognition of realities beyond those that can be observed with our five senses. These are grounded mainly in nonscientific, although not antiscientific, evidences (Moberg, 1967).

For example, the question of what life is leads to the conclusion that it is more than the sum of the identifiable parts of biological organisms. Processes indicate that life is present, but it is more than processes alone. The totality of a person somehow resides in his or her spiritual nature, not in the conglomeration of separate parts and processes that can be abstracted from reality for analysis in research laboratories.

Similarly, human beings are autonomous and cannot be reduced to completely determined creatures that are only puppets of their genetic and cultural heritage. The human spirit transcends the material elements of the world. Through the mind, it imposes "reality" on intangible phenomena such as space and time. Each person is self-conscious, develops self-concepts, sees one's self as a unity, and distinguishes self from everyone else, and has the capacity for decision making, an inherent quality that is a core feature of one's spiritual personhood.

In addition, each person has subjective experiences that are distinct from objective reality, as refelected in the "other minds" problem of philosophy. Apart from using electrocardiographic or other technical equipment, a person can only observe and study the externalized responses of another person to such mental states as love, faith, or pain. One cannot "know" the internalized reponses.

Likewise, knowing things about a person is not the same as knowing a person. Two or more people who intimately share mutual experiences and knowledge of each other may enter into a relationship with experiences of oneness that is similar to the spiritual relationship of a devout person with God.

Numerous "proofs" for the existence of God and the belief that all people are related to God, positively or negatively, have been developed in theological apologetics. People who choose to believe find a wealth of resources to support their faith, which includes belief in the supernatural essence and spirituality of humanity.

Evidence for the ontological reality of the spiritual nature of humanity is circumstantial, philosophical, existential, and theological; hence, it is inconclusive for positivists who insist that scientific criteria of empirical sensory observations are the only acceptable basis for reality and truth. The evidence is, however, strongly supported by the history of both preliterate and world religions, which also suggests that most, if not all, people have an innate desire for a spiritual commitment or all-embracing concern to which they can give personal loyalty. Even those early sociologists who believed traditional religions should be eradicated recognized society's need for an integrating faith, so they substituted an ideology of science and education.

The dominant source of spiritual instruction in Western civilization has been the Bible. It remains the most significant "textbook" on the subject and is accepted by a large majority of older adults in America as the most authoritative resource on spirituality and aging.

SPIRITUALITY AND AGING
IN THE BIBLE

The Bible begins with the words, "In the beginning God [Hebrew *Elohim*] created the heavens and the earth. Now the earth was formless and empty, darkness was over the surface of the deep, and the Spirit [Hebrew *ruach*] of God was hovering over the waters" (Genesis 1:1-2, NIV). The plural-form name for God, *Elohim,* appears approximately 2,300 times and *Yahweh* ["the Existing One"], usually translated as *Jehovah* or *LORD,* about 4,300 times (Young, 1974). God is presented as the eternally existent Creator who is named simply "I AM" (Exodus 3:14).

Then "God created man in his own image, in the image of God he created him; male and female he created them" (Genesis 1:27, NIV). They became a living soul *[nephesh]* when God breathed the breath of life into them (Genesis 2:7). Centuries later Jesus said, "God is spirit [Greek *pneuma*], and his worshipers must worship in spirit and in truth" (John 4:24, NIV). God "set eternity in the hearts of men" (Ecclesiastes 3:11, NIV). These and other passages clearly indicate the consistent biblical truth that the essence of humanity is not the body but the spirit and soul, words that often are interchangeable although not necessarily synonyms. They are flexible and imprecise terms in the Bible, not intended to provide highly technical distinctions from each other (see Reymond, 1998, pp. 415-457).

The Hebrew *ruach* and Greek *pneuma,* most often translated as spirit, appear hundreds of times in the Bible, as do the words *nephish* and *psuche* that usually are translated as soul. The soul is not something separate from the body but rather the total person (Whitlock, 1983). In the Bible the spiritual nature of humanity is simply taken for granted and is implied in numerous passages without those words. Over the past generation there have been

> ... strong trends within psychology to resurrect man *in toto* from a misplaced emphasis on him [sic] as a compound of variables and fractionated processes. Current humanistic-psychological versions of man *qua* man are basically similar to the views of man held in Western theology. (Spilka, 1983, p. 79)

The Hebrew prophets, Jesus, and New Testament apostles often called for a genuinely spiritual, God-honoring faith that stood in stark contrast to hypocritical repetition of traditional religious practices. They strongly condemned persons who drew near to God only with their mouths, honoring him with words but with unjust deeds and hearts far removed from him (e.g., Isaiah 29:13-21; James 1:22-27).

References to spirituality (spiritual blessings, discernment, food, gifts, persons, sacrifices, songs, truths, wickedness, wisdom, etc.) are sprinkled throughout the Bible. The hope of resurrection after death for those who trust their redeemer (Job 19:25-27; 1 Corinthians 15:42-58) helps believers stand firm in their faith and live the kind of life that pleases God (Romans 12:1-2). The promises of Scripture elevate the self-images of believers, strengthen their ability to transcend the limitations and losses of aging, and give power to cope realistically with disability, suffering, and other problems that may come their way (see Stagg, 1981; Koenig, 1994).

IS SPIRITUALITY JUST ANOTHER WORD FOR RELIGION?

Religion

The claim has been made that no major human society has been without a religion, at least not until modern Western civilization. The diminishing levels of membership in churches, synagogues, and other religious organizations, along with the slowly increasing proportions of adults in America and Europe who claim to be agnostics or atheists, suggest that modern Western civilization may be moving toward religionlessness. Yet some interpreters of contemporary cultures believe that even secularists who profess they have no religion are actually "worshiping" gods of technology, materialism ("mammon"), sex, or self-adoration, and thus have a religion of their own.

One could easily compile a list with dozens of definitions of religion. Most can be categorized under one or more of the following four types:

1. *Belief in supernatural power, force, or beings, accompanied by efforts to get into and remain in a favorable relationship with it or them.* This includes some form of dependence upon supernatural or nonnatural powers.
2. *Belief in values that are thought to transcend immediate social circumstances, and therefore to be worthy of allegiance.* Sometimes described as "a set of ultimate meanings and values expressed in a creed," this includes the symbols, activities, and organizations that promote and sustain such values.
3. *Systems of beliefs and values that explain the mysterious and the unknown or answer teleological questions (those dealing with meaning, final or ultimate causes, and purposes).* This includes the social organizations into which the beliefs and values have been incorporated.
4. *The sacralization of identity, a process of making sacred whatever reinforces social order and harnesses change.* Through mechanisms of objectification, commitment, ritual, and myth this provides order, anchors emotions, reinforces rites, and consolidates beliefs (Mol, 1976, 1983).

Within religious institutions and groups, however large or small, are members who have varying degrees of intensity and commitment. Ideally, their congregations, along with subsidiary fellowship, service, prayer, or study groups, reinforce beliefs, promote worship, engage in rituals, support service projects and ministries, help members share their faith with others without forcing it upon them, and foster ideals of living consistently with their beliefs and values. But members with little or no true or intrinsic religious commitment cannot easily be separated from those of deep faith and loyalty, so the hypocrisy of negative associations of conduct with religiousness is common.

Organizational and group activities related to a system of faith and worship are easily observed and therefore are a central focus of attention in references to religion, under which the spiritual domain usually has been implicitly subsumed. Research on religion has often used simplistic one-dimensional indicators or "measures." Among these are a person's religious membership or nonmembership, frequency of attending religious activities, family religious heritage, and religious or nonreligious self-identification. Crude as the measures using single categories are, many personal and social characteristics have been found to be associated with them, often in surprising relationships. Lenski (1961) discovered that the impact of religion on the daily lives of people in modern society, and through them upon other institutional systems of their communities (especially economics, politics, education, and family life), is far more significant than that of many favorite sociological research variables. Similar findings have emerged repeatedly from social scientific studies of religion.

Nevertheless, the generalizations about religion expressed by scholars and social scientists often contradict each other for many reasons: (1) religious beliefs and behavior are very diverse; (2) people tend to extend conclusions based upon one or more religious persons or groups to all religions; (3) the definitions of religion used in research vary widely and are not necessarily consistent with each other; (4) the measures and indicators of religiousness used in research are extremely numerous and diverse; (5) the methods and techniques used in research on religion are numerous, each viewing its object of study from a somewhat different perspective; (6) those methods are sometimes biased as a result of conscious or unconscious values of the researchers, the manner in which the persons or groups investigated are sampled, the selection of questions asked and topics explored, the theoretical frame of reference adopted, response categories that the researcher thinks are important, limited sharing of information because of the taken-for-granted nature of insiders' views, the relative secrecy of some "inside" behavior and experience (e.g., "gentiles" kept out of Mormon temples), and the halo effect when persons investigated reveal themselves in a more favorable religious light than is true of their actual beliefs and conduct (professed ideals versus actual attitudes and behavior); and (7) there are many ways to interpret and report research findings. As a result, the same data may be used both in an argument favoring a specific generalization or religious group and in one opposing it. Opposite impressions can be conveyed simply by the insertion of an adjective in a report. For example, the weekly attendance at religious services reported in public opinion polls of U.S. adults can be contrasted with their religious membership of nearly two-thirds of the population as "only 40 percent" or by comparisons with other nations "a surprisingly high 40 percent."

Spirituality

Spirituality is tightly interwoven with religion. It is rarely understood in religiously neutral terms, however, although interpretations of it as denoting "an individual's or community's ultimate existential aspirations and the means of achieving these aspirations" (Kirkwood, 1994, p. 16) may seem nonreligious because they are not theistically oriented and do not mention God. Throughout human history, and apparently even during prehistoric eras, people have given much attention to spiritual phenomena. This has taken many forms, including the following:

- Calling upon mediums and spirit guides for spiritual discernment, fortune telling, and divination in decision making, especially by kings and chieftains.
- Real or alleged possession by spirits, whether for good or ill.
- Beliefs in nontheistic animist religions that all things have spirits.
- Encounters with and worship of the Deity, spirits, the Great Spirit, or gods.
- Human or other sacrifices to one or more gods, as among the Ancient Hebrews, the Mayans in Central America, and offerings of flowers, fruit, chickens, etc. by many Buddhists and Hindus.
- Attributing human fate, weather, and other events to the actions or will of Norse, Greek, Roman, Babylonian, or other gods.

The definition of spirituality that was used in the landmark Spiritual Well-Being Section of the 1971 White House Conference on Aging centered around people's inner resources, especially their "ultimate concern, the basic value around which all other values are focused, the central philosophy of life—whether religious, antireligious, or nonreligious—which guides a person's conduct, the supernatural and nonmaterial dimensions of human nature" (Moberg, 1971, p. 3). The importance of direct attention to meeting people's spiritual needs was a central concern as that section formulated and recommended fourteen types of action (see White House Conference on Aging, 1971; Chapter 14, this volume).

Many complications of communication about spirituality flow out of the great diversity of religious and ideological traditions. Even within each monotheistic religion (especially Judaism, Islam, and Christianity), there are many forms of spirituality. In Eastern religions, new religious movements based upon them, and even some Christian groups spirituality refers to a denial of reality, seclusion or withdrawal from "the world," the nonbeing of nirvana, consciousness of "the god that is within you," or other forms of philosophical idealism. Some strands of such thought have a wholly inward orientation, stressing warm experiential feelings of interiorized spirituality while neutralizing the social conscience or making materialism a pejorative term as people try to escape from hard realities of the world (Leech, 1986).

Lane (1984) has identified four aspects of the Christian spiritual life:

1. A Christian outlook that is "a reflex, intellectual faith-vision of the world"
2. Finding or seeking God in contemplation and prayer
3. Finding God in activity that makes prayer a style of life in God's service
4. The "experiential awareness of the presence of God" that is a special gift of sensing God's operative presence in the world and in oneself (pp. 74-76)

Persons and communities that are firmly rooted in personal experience with God are empowered to become committed, creative forces for transforming society, so individualism is held in balance with social consciousness (Sears, 1984).

In popular culture, countless magazine articles, pamphlets, books, and videos offer inspirational interpretations and advice on how to deepen and enrich spirituality. Retreats and workshops, sermons and lectures, conferences and seminars, literature and the arts, and movies and dramas, set forth disparate views about how to stimulate and cultivate personal peace with oneself, others, the universe, or God. Some expound conventional goals of inspiring and deepening faith, sensing the wonder of the Creator's handiwork, reflecting and reminiscing upon God's goodness and mercy, and attaining salvation or feelings of shalom and oneness with the Deity or universe. Others emphasize techniques of guided imagery, relaxation formulas, physical exercises, dietary cleansing, herbalism, astrology, mantra chanting, meditation, dancing, or myriads of other rituals as the means for "spiritual renewal" or attaining "total well-being of body, mind, and spirit." Anyone trying to keep up with all of "the latest" approaches to spirituality is bound to get confused.

PERCEPTIONS OF SPIRITUALITY AND RELIGION

Research has shown that most Americans have rather definite ideas about the characteristics associated with, influencing, and affected by spirituality and spiritual wellness, even though they have difficulty defining such concepts (Moberg, 1979). Some refer to subjective feeling states like inner peace, serenity, or self-actualization. Many describe the essential characteristics in religious terms like peace with God or faith in Jesus Christ. Others emphasize social relationships like helping others, having faith in people, being a participating member of a religious congregation or spiritual family, or living a moral and ethical life. Most believe that spirituality gives meaning to life, aids in decision making, and is a necessary component of health through faith in oneself, in life after death, in a supreme being, or even in the goodness of all people. Few describe it in terms of material prosperity or social respectability, although most believe that spiritual wellness contributes to economic success but that the wealthy are no more likely than the poor to be spiritually well.

A study by Zinnbauer and colleagues (1997) of how 346 individuals define religiousness and spirituality, their self-ratings of those qualities, and correlations with predictor variables and other self-characterizations resulted in three main conclusions. (1) The terms describe different concepts and have different correlates. *Religiousness* includes both personal beliefs (as in God) and organizational practices like church activities and commitment to the belief system of a religion. It is associated with higher levels of authoritarianism, religious orthodoxy, parental religious attendance, self-righteousness, and church attendance. *Spirituality* is most often described in experiential terms such as faith in God or a higher power or integrating one's values and beliefs with behavior in daily life. It sometimes is associated with mystical experiences and New Age beliefs and practices. (2) Although religiousness and spirituality describe different concepts, they are modestly but significantly correlated, not totally independent. Most people consider themselves to be both religious and spiritual. Their self-rated religiousness and spirituality are associated with frequency of prayer, church attendance, religious orthodoxy, and an intrinsic religiosity that uses religion as a guiding point for everyday decisions. (3) Although 93 percent identify themselves as spiritual, some rate themselves high on spirituality and low on religion, while others are moderate on both. Thus most believers approach the sacred through the personal, subjective, and experiential path of spirituality, even though they differ on whether they should include organizational or institutional beliefs and practices in their self-identity.

RESOLVING DEFINITIONAL CONFUSION

The diverse and confusing interpretations of spirituality in today's society are also evident in professional practice and scientific research. Many of the dilemmas related to understanding and analyzing spirituality can be resolved by an analogy to physical life, maturity, and health. Babies need almost two decades to attain physical maturity, while their personality development, character growth, and progression toward social, occupational, marital, and other forms of maturity may continue for several more decades.

Yet one's existence does not depend upon whether one is healthy or ill. A person may have different degrees of physical wellness at each stage of life. If the body is healthy in all organs except one, we tend to focus upon the imperfection and label a person who is, say, "95 percent well," as sick or disabled. All of the body's hundreds of parts and processes are interrelated and influence each other, but each can be analyzed as if on a scale from perfectly well, then mostly well, and then partly, mostly, or totally ill. Similar evaluations of mental health and illness compound the formula for total wellness.

Since the essence of every person is spirit, every body is spiritual. There are, however, relative degrees of spiritual maturity and immaturity, as well as of spiritual wellness and illness. Each dimension and component of spirituality can be evaluated separately, yielding intricate, interacting entanglements of the types and degrees of spiritual health and maturity. When these are combined with the complex components of physical and mental health, the picture of total well-being or wholistic health that emerges is of such incredible complexity that it defies our imaginations. Nevertheless, as we shall see in Chapter 4, considerable research is already probing the ways in which spirituality interacts with physical and mental health.

A wholistic approach to understanding human wellness focuses less upon its countless analytically separable physical, mental, and spiritual dimensions than upon how they all come together and cannot be separated in real life. (Incidentally, I prefer the *wholistic* spelling because *holistic* ideals often omit the spiritual domain or reduce it to psychiatric and other variables, thus leaving a hole in what ought to be kept whole.) If we agree that the essence of each person is spirit, then "the role of the spiritual is to be an integrative element in the life of the individual, . . . not one dimension, but an integrative dimension" (Ellor and Bracki, 1995, p. 155).

Individuals may or may not be aware of their true spiritual condition. Like a seemingly healthy person whose body has a hidden cancer that is metastasizing to other organs without giving pain or other symptoms, some who are inflicted with an unrecognized spiritual malignancy, flaw, or disease may wrongly think they are spiritually well. Others may erroneously believe they are ill during "dark night of the soul" experiences that stimulate their spiritual development. Many have sufficient resources (faith in God, friends, significant others, clergy, spiritual counselors, the Scriptures, etc.) to correctly evaluate their spiritual health and maturity. Appropriate professional resources can assist individuals in attaining a more accurate spiritual diagnosis than they would have without such help.

The criteria currently used to evaluate spirituality usually come from an ideological, theoretical, or theological source. Thus in a Christian frame of reference, believers trust Bible promises that they possess eternal spiritual life through Jesus Christ by virtue of God's unmerited favor (grace), not by their own achievements. They are warned in passages such as 1 John 1:8-10 that if they claim to be without sin, they deceive themselves and do not tell the truth. Although only God knows with absolute certainty the degree to which each is spiritually well or ill, the Bible emphasizes that spiritual growth is a lifelong pursuit, and it includes many criteria (e.g., "acts of the sinful nature" and "fruit of the Spirit" [Galatians 5:14-26, NIV]) for evaluating Christian spiritual health and maturity. Parallel reference points, principles, and criteria for assessing spirituality are found in most other religions.

The evaluative criteria used in research, however, seldom come directly from Christian or other theologies and sacred writings. They more often are derived from theories of disciplines like psychology and sociology or from assumptions and postulates that undergird the clinical work of counselors, mental health professionals, and clergy.

Each profession has its own specialized foci of attention and values, but also competing schools of thought and practice. The research of some aims to discover relationships between spirituality and other phenomena. Others develop diagnostic tools for helping people spiritually or tests for determining whether or not programs, services, and other interventions to enhance spirituality are effective. As a result, the specific components of spirituality scales vary widely even when they carry similar labels, such as spiritual well-being.

Spiritual Well-Being (SWB)

Soon after the National Interfaith Coalition on Aging (NICA) was organized as a by-product of the 1971 WHCA, it surveyed ministries with and for the aging. It quickly discovered that its Protestant, Catholic, and Jewish agencies had a wide range of implicit definitions of spirituality, so in 1975 it convened an interdisciplinary interfaith workshop to deal with the problem. It concluded that NICA should use a one-sentence "working-with" definition:

> Spiritual well-being is the affirmation of life in a relationship with God, self, community, and environment that nurtures and celebrates wholeness. (NICA, 1975)

NICA's commentary explained, "The spiritual is not one dimension among many in life; rather, it permeates and gives meaning to all life. The term spiritual well-being, therefore, indicates wholeness in contrast to fragmentation and isolation" (Thorson and Cook, 1980, p. xiii).

NICA's (1975) pragmatic definition has been adapted for use in a wide variety of theologies, traditions, and linguistic communities. It has been a useful stimulus for professional practice among those who wish to include spirituality in clinical work or to evaluate programs designed to serve whole-person spiritual needs. Nevertheless, it has not appealed to researchers in the scientific study of spirituality because each of its major concepts (affirmation, life, relationship, community, environment, nurtures, celebrates, wholeness) is subject to extremely diverse interpretations.

Scientific research on spirituality has narrowed the vast subject by identifying and measuring variables related to the health or maturity of the human spirit. Dozens of implicit and explicit definitions of spiritual well-being (SWB) are found, for instance, even in a single collection of articles by twenty-seven sociologists (Moberg, 1979). Some represent relatively conventional Christian interpretations of a meaningful, purposeful relationship with God that influences one's relationships with people. Others assume the foundation of SWB is the need of persons and groups to transcend themselves or that SWB is a never-ending process of becoming while one occupies the role-set of membership in a religious organization. The evidences of SWB used include healthy self-concepts, faith, belief in the bigness of God, unselfish giving to others, following the lifestyle of Jesus, finding satisfaction in religion, intrinsic religiousness, coming to terms with sin, and moral character (Moberg, 1979). All of these may be specific components or correlates of spiritual health, but hundreds, if not thousands, of additional indicators also could be used to reflect or measure SWB.

Like alienation, intelligence, loneliness, and many other concepts in the social and behavioral sciences, spirituality is intangible, identifiable only through indirect observation and an artificially abstracted breakdown of its component parts and dimensions. Again by analogy, we cannot see personality, yet it is described and defined by selected traits and characteristics, such as intraversion-extroversion, integrity-nondependability, and deceptiveness-honesty, each of which has subdimensions on which a person may score high or low. The overall personality assessment depends upon which specific traits are included and which components are observed for each trait.

Similarly, the results of research on spirituality depend upon the components included. Every instrument to measure or evaluate SWB or spiritual maturity consists of its own set of indicators and therefore is, in effect, a unique "operational definition"—one based upon, and thus defined by, the information sought and questions asked through the interviews, observations, and other evidence that contribute to the assessment (see Chapter 15). When attributes and variables interpreted by one frame of reference or scale to be signs or indicators of spiritual wellness are considered to be symptoms of spiritual illness by another, our analytical and interpretive skills are challenged. Presumably, the expanding variety of scales and investigative techniques enriches our understanding of spiritual well-being.

CONCLUSIONS

Historically, spirituality was seldom distinguished from religion, and both were considered to have mixed positive and negative elements and consequences. By the 1960s and 1970s, under the impact of increasing popular disillusionment with religious institutions, *spirituality* began to acquire meanings and connotations that separated it from religion. It gained more positive than negative connotations through its association with personal experiences of the transcendent, while *religiousness* has tended to have more negative than positive connotations, partly because of connections with institutional religion, which some view as a hindrance to such experiences. *Spirituality* now is an "in" word, even among groups such as the baby boomers who defected from conventional religions and turned to New Age movements that emphasize direct spiritual experience and claim to be spiritual but not religious. They tend to be more individualistic, to engage in mystical religious beliefs and practices, to view their faith as a spiritual journey or quest, and to hold nontheistic beliefs about God (see Roof, 1993).

Until recently *religion* and *religiousness* included both individual and institutional elements, but now they often are identified with formally structured religious institutions that typically advocate prescribed theologies and rituals. Many concerns of organized religion (maintaining properties, paying bills, supervising staff, scheduling meetings, organizing and managing group activities, etc.) are not primarily spiritual except in terms of their leaders' and members' motivations, commitments, and goals.

Yet awakening, nurturing, and deepening the spirituality of people—enhancing their spiritual well-being and maturity—ideally is the central goal or purpose beneath religious rituals, activities, and organizational structures. *Spirituality,* therefore, is usually regarded as a subjective personal phenomenon that is identified with such things as faith commitments, behavior consistent with beliefs, personal transcendence, supraconscious sensitivity, and meaningfulness.

Spirituality has many subdimensions, so we must be very careful not to evaluate the spiritual health and maturity of others superficially or carelessly. That precaution is especially important among human service professionals who may have influence and power over other people. Therapy, research, communication, and often people's feelings of life satisfaction and well-being, as well as their actual spiritual health, can all suffer from inconsistent understandings of spirituality or defective means to enhance it.

Every person has existence as a living soul or spirit and thus has spirituality, but each experiences varying levels of spiritual health and spiritual maturity.

> Spiritual well-being could, indeed, be the true awareness, the true happiness, the true purposiveness, and the true freedom— the pearl without price for which all other things can profitably be exchanged. And it might be found that many who are abundantly endowed with other things, even things closely associated with it, know very little of it. (Fallding, 1979, p. 40)

But all who read on in this book will gain an increased awareness and understanding of the nature of spirituality and its significance for personal and professional life in the complex world of which we are a part.

REFERENCES

Bailey, Edward (1998). "Implicit religion": What might that be? *Implicit Religion* 1(November):9-22.

Cimino, Richard and Don Lattin (1999). Choosing my religion. *American Demographics* 21(4):62-65.

Ellor, James W. and Marie A. Bracki (1995). Assessment, referral, and networking. In Kimble, M. A., S. H. McFadden, J. W. Ellor, and J. J. Seeber (Eds.), *Aging, spirituality, and religion: A handbook* (pp. 148-160). Minneapolis, MN: Fortress Press.

Fallding, Harold (1979). Spiritual well-being as a variety of good morale. In Moberg, David O. (Ed.), *Spiritual well-being: Sociological perspectives* (pp. 23-40). Washington, DC: University Press of America.

Gallup, George (1999). Assessing religion in U.S. on three levels. *Emerging Trends* 21(3):2-4.

Kirkwood, William G. (1994). Studying communication about spirituality and the spiritual consequences of communication. *Journal of Communication and Religion* 17(1):13-16.

Koenig, Harold G. (1994). Religion and hope for the disabled elder. In Levin, Jeffrey S. (Ed.), *Religion in aging and health* (pp. 18-51). Thousand Oaks, CA: Sage Publications.

Koenig, Harold G. (1997). *Is religion good for your health?* Binghamton, NY: The Haworth Press.

Lane, George A. (1984). *Christian spirituality—An historical sketch.* Chicago: Loyola University Press.

Leech, Kenneth (1986). The soul and the social order. *Weavings* 1(2):6-13.

Lenski, Gerhard (1961). *The religious factor: A sociological study of religion's impact on politics, economics, and family life.* Garden City, NY: Doubleday & Co.

Lentini, Alison (1999). Lost in the supermarket: Pop music and spiritual commerce. *SCP Journal* 22(4) and 23(1):18-25.

Moberg, David O. (1967). The encounter of scientific and religious values pertinent to man's spiritual nature. *Sociological Analysis* 28(1):22-33.

Moberg, David O. (1971). *Spiritual well-being: Background and issues.* Washington, DC: White House Conference on Aging.

Moberg, David O. (1979). The development of social indicators of spiritual well-being for quality of life research. In Moberg, David O. (Ed.), *Spiritual well-being: Sociological perspectives* (pp. 1-13). Washington, DC: University Press of America.

Mol, Johannis (Hans) J. (1976). *Identity and the sacred.* Oxford: Blackwell.

Mol, Johannis (Hans) J. (1983). *Meaning and place: An introduction to the social scientific study of religion.* New York: The Pilgrim Press.

NICA (1975). *Spiritual well-being.* Athens, GA: National Interfaith Coalition on Aging.

NIV: *The Holy Bible,* New International Version (1984). Colorado Springs, CO: International Bible Society.

Reymond, Robert (1998). *Systematic theology of the Christian faith.* Irving, TX: Word Books.

Roof, Wade Clark (1993). *A generation of seekers: The spiritual journeys of the baby boom generation.* San Francisco: HarperCollins.

Sears, Robert T. (1984). Afterword. In Lane, George A. (Ed.), *Christian spirituality* (pp. 77-80). Chicago: Loyola University Press.

Spilka, Bernard (1983). Images of man and dimensions of personal religion: Values for an empirical psychology of religion. In Malony, H. Newton (Ed.), *Wholeness and holiness: Readings in the psychology/theology of mental health* (pp. 67-82). Grand Rapids, MI: Baker Book Co.

Stagg, Frank (1981). *The Bible speaks on aging.* Nashville, TN: Broadman Press.

Sturzo, Luigi (1947). *The true life: Sociology of the supernatural* (B.B. Carter, translator). London: Geoffrey Bles.

Thorson, James A. and Thomas C. Cook, Jr. (Eds.). (1980). *Spiritual well-being of the elderly.* Springfield, IL: Charles C Thomas.

Van Kaam, Adrian L. (1992). *Formative spirituality, Volume 5: Traditional formation.* New York: Crossroad Publishing Co.

White House Conference on Aging (1971). *Section recommendations on spiritual well-being.* Washington, DC: Government Printing Office.

Whitlock, Glenn E. (1983). The structure of personality in Hebrew psychology. In Malony, H. Newton (Ed.), *Wholeness and holiness: Readings in the psychology/theology of mental health* (pp. 41-51). Grand Rapids, MI: Baker Book Co.

Wuthnow, Robert (1998). *After heaven: Spirituality in America since the 1950s.* Berkeley: University of California Press.

Young, Robert (1974). *Analytical concordance to the Bible, 22nd American edition.* Grand Rapids, MI: Eerdmans.

Zinnbauer, Brian J., Kenneth I. Pargament, Brenda Cole, Mark S. Rye, Eric M. Butter, Timothy G. Belavich, Kathleen M. Hipp, Allie B. Scott, and Jill L. Kadar (1997). Religion and spirituality: Unfuzzying the fuzzy. *Journal for the Scientific Study of Religion* 36(4):549-564.

Chapter 2

The Spiritual Role of the Elder in the Twenty-First Century

Robert J. Best

It is no secret that unprecedented numbers of Americans are living long into the period we call old age. People are enjoying better health and are better educated than ever before (Griffin,1997), yet our society continues to have a very unfavorable attitude toward aging. People in our culture try to avoid or deny the aging process, and the term elder is anything but a title of honor.

Although ageism is a complex and multifaceted problem, one of the reasons so many people dread the onset of elderhood is that society has failed to develop meaningful roles for older adults in families and communities. As people age, they move through a series of socially structured roles, from student to worker, from single person to spouse, from individual to parent (Riley and Waring, 1978). The transition from one role to another can be difficult and painful. However, "role transitions can be positive experiences when the new role is socially valued and when people provide adequate social and emotional support during the transition"(Riley and Waring, 1978, p. 64). In contemporary American culture, the role of elder is essentially nonexistent, let alone socially valued, with little social or emotional support available.

PAST ROLES FOR ELDERS

The lack of roles for elders is a relatively new phenomenon. A look at the roots of most cultures reveals a long history of important and valued roles for elders. This is evident throughout the world but is particularly true in the Asian, African, Native American, and Hispanic cultures. In these earlier cultures, elders were considered essential to the continuity and identity of the community. In ancient Israel, elders performed deliberative, representative, and judicial functions and were admitted to that governing body purely on the basis of age (Campbell, 1994, p. 22).

Recognizing the unique gifts that came with advanced age, the community expected the elders to contribute to the vitality and spiritual well-being of the younger members. Responsible elders carefully scrutinized the progress and behavior of the young. It was to the elders that the young came for permission to move toward adulthood (Cox and Mberia, 1975, p. 3).

One of the roles of the elder was that of *Repository of Wisdom*. This role was the result of the recognition that elders have increased knowledge by virtue of their years of living (Wimberly, 1997, p. 8). People may argue that, in the past as today, not all older people have wisdom. However, the people of earlier times realized that there was something about the lives of older adults, whether tragic or hopeful, from which younger people could learn and find guidance. This is sometimes referred to as practical wisdom, or in some African cultures as "mother wit." It is an intuitive knowledge of how to judge a situation and what to do (Wimberly, 1997, p. 8). Younger people turned to the elders for counsel and advice during difficult or confusing times.

Elders also function in the community as *Celebrators of Rituals*. In the Japanese culture, the older people were the primary perpetuators of religious affairs (Palmore, 1975, p. 45). Elders made offerings and participated in private devotions and communal prayer on behalf of the entire family or community. They had a visible role in liturgical celebrations and religious ceremonies.

Elders usually played a special role in the spiritual education of young people. They were *Transmitters of Sacred Knowledge* (Wall, 1993). They taught the young about the scriptures and myths of their culture. In many communities, it was the work of the elders to teach young people how to pray (Wimberly, 1997, p. 10).

The elders were revered for their historical significance. They were seen as *Conduits to the Past*. Their very presence created a connection between generations past, present, and future. They established an awareness of the culture and the rootedness that was so necessary for the health and growth of the community.

LOSS OF VALUE
FOR THE ROLE OF ELDER

During the Industrial Age, the roles for older people became distorted and American culture lost sight of their importance. There were a variety of reasons for this deterioration in the importance of elders.

With the advent of the manufacturing model, American society began to place ever-increasing emphasis on material production. People began to measure the value of actions by criteria of efficiency and material success (Pontifical Council for the Laity, 1999, p. 8). Older peoples' reduced ability to produce material goods led to an undervaluing of the altruistic role of the elder. As Percy (1974) described it almost three decades ago:

> We value productivity. If someone is not "productive" (is that word to be measured only in terms of Gross National Product?) he or she has little value. . . . Too often, that is precisely our attitude toward the aged in America. (p. 2)

The Industrial Age brought with it an exaggerated appreciation for science and technology and a skepticism for intuition and accumulated experience. Knowledge gained from science and technology seemed to supplant the value of knowledge gained from experience (Pontifical Council for the Laity, 1999). Modern writers have suggested that

> Industrialization and rapid social change have transformed the aged into cast-out, useless relics of the past who are a burden at best and are often a nuisance and obstruction to modern progress and enlightenment. (Palmore, 1975, p. 3)

Another phenomenon that tends to diminish the role of elders is cultural surrender. Cultural surrender is the process whereby people fail to take time to learn the heritage of parents or ancestors (Cox and Mberia, 1975, p. 3). As a result, generations lose a sense of history and, consequently, a sense of their own identity. It diminishes the possibility of learning positive parenting and grandparenting roles.

Closely related to the process of cultural surrender is the concept of individualism. It involves an emphasis on self-seeking behavior and often leads to abandonment of the weaker members of the community (Pontifical Council for the Laity, 1999, p. 8). The result, once again, is a lack of value for older adults.

Another side effect of the industrial age that presents an obstacle to the role of elders is the segregation of generations. Bly (1990, p. 45) refers to sibling communities, in which people are exposed to and interact with only members of their own age group. As a result, they seek "substitute wisdoms" from peers and the media, rather than looking to elder mentors (Wimberly, 1997, p. 9).

At first glance, the idea of segregation of generations would seem to be an argument against older people's living in or forming their own retirement communities. This, however, is not necessarily the case. There may be good reasons, both practical and spiritual, for older adults to live together, apart from the younger generations.

More and more older people have discovered that the later years can prove to be the most favorable time of all for spiritual development (Griffin, 1997). Many often feel the need to devote more time and energy to prayer and other spiritual practices in an effort to find stronger meaning in their lives. Like the monasteries of the middle ages, retirement communities could represent a place where older adults gather to live in community, reflect on their lives, and share their common experiences. These communities could be great centers of learning and contemplation. They could become places where culture, knowledge, and beauty are preserved, as the European monasteries did during the Barbarian invasions.

Unfortunately, today's retirement communities place undue emphasis on activity and very little on contemplation. There is no arena for elders to share their stories, visions, and dreams. Even more tragic is the lack of opportunity for people living in these communities to discuss their insights with younger people. Many retirement communities lack the sense of hospitality, which was an important part of the monastic movement.

It is possible to imagine a retirement community that encourages and teaches its members to spend time in meditation, prayer, and reflection. It would provide focused opportunities for members to learn from each other and to make connections between their life stories, the stories of their religious traditions, and the stories of others within the community.

This monastic-type retirement community would also need to reach out to the other generations. It could become a retreat center for people of all ages who are seeking spiritual growth and a deeper understanding of life. The members of the community would need to strengthen their skills at hospitality, and make it inviting to others.

RECLAIMING THE ROLE OF ELDER

What should be the role of the elder today and in the future? The later years of life should be a time to develop the interior life, imagination, intellect, and judgment. They can be a time to become more appreciative, more contemplative, more prayerful (Fahey, 1987). But, they also are a time to become more deeply involved with others, both with individuals and with society as a whole. As Eugene Bianchi (1990) describes this:

> Emphasis on interiority should not suggest withdrawal from the world in elderhood. Rather, the interior life becomes, in part, a preparation for contributing the authentic wisdom of age to the central concerns of communities and nations. (p. 208)

The potential roles for the elders of today are similar to the roles of days gone by. However, these same roles take on a slightly different flavor in our modern world.

One important role for the elder in modern society is that of *Storyteller/Historian.* The elder can help to preserve history and make the past come alive for succeeding generations. According to Pipher (1999): "Americans are losing our cultural memory. We have short attention spans and live in the eternal now of advertising. Elders can help with this" (p. 12). Elders are the memory of the community and the "living library" of history (Wimberly, 1997, p. 28). A society that ignores the past can easily run the risk of repeating its mistakes (Pontifical Council for the Laity, 1999).

Elders tell the stories of how things were and where we are all coming from. They tell stories growing out of real lived experience. This gives younger people a broader view of life so they are no longer dependent solely upon their own time and culture to define reality. "The outlook of another generation gives us what is called 'social immunity,' an independence of thought and values" (Boucher, 1991, p. 72). Stories have a transforming impact upon both the listener and the teller.

Historical events are important, whether they relate to world history or family history. Each family needs pieces of oral tradition to help its members get their bearings (Boucher, 1991, p. 72). If the elder has reflected on the ultimate meaning of events and relationships, then personal history can have a deeply spiritual dimension. The values and attitudes that past experiences have engendered in the storyteller become evident to others (Boucher, 1991). Storytelling is richest when it comes from a person who has lived a full life and has reflected on those experiences (Wilhelm, 1987).

Elders have great potential to invite the generations to come together as *Gatherers of Family/Community.* Even with our often hurried lifestyles, families tend to gather around the older members (usually women), and they count on the elders to provide the glue that binds the family together. There is extensive literature showing that older women are the "kin-keepers," and that they start preparation for this role very early in life.

> Kin-keeping tasks include maintaining communication, facilitating contact and the exchange of goods and services, and monitoring family relationships. These functions are often performed for both the husband's kin as well as for the woman's own family line. Even when they are not initiators and orchestrators of family get-togethers, old women may nevertheless facilitate family contact by serving as the "excuse" for bringing kin together. (Hagestad, 1986, p. 150)

Elders have a role even if they have no grandchildren of their own or grandchildren are geographically separated. "All children need to be grandchildren and all elders need to be grandparents. We all need more hugs, laughs, and stories" (Wilhelm, 1987, p. 4). Elders can be grandparents for the neighborhood. But, to be such, they must learn hospitality and playfulness.

The role of the elder is different and complementary to that of parent. Elders tend to have less responsibility than parents in the areas of task performance, discipline, and problem solving, but in the area of comfort and affectional support, elders can be most important (Palmore, 1975, p. 46). Sometimes, children need an advocate in the face of parental power. Children may find it difficult to deal with the power of their parents, physically, psychologically, and emotionally.

There is a need for an elder with wisdom, advice, consolation, and advocacy (Wilhelm, 1987). Elders can provide a place of mercy beyond justice. They have learned that, in the long run, it is not really possible to control others or to make decisions for them. "Without undermining parental authority, elders can balance the uneven scales of power between parents and children" (Wilhelm, 1987, p. 3).

Our contemporary culture is sorely lacking in *Mentors and Role Models*. Elders can educate younger people about the successes and mistakes they have made, and what they have learned in the process. They remind younger people of core values and why they are values. As people age and lose physical strength and vitality, they learn to live more quietly and more simply. Young people need to learn this lesson. As Father Eschweiler (1999), a retired pastor, put it, "They value quality over quantity in activities and relationships, with other people and with God. They learn to clarify what is important and what is really not." The Pontifical Council on the Laity (1999) states:

> The affective, moral and religious values embodied by older people are an indispensable resource for fostering the harmony of society, of the family and the individual. These values include a sense of responsibility, faith in God, friendship, disinterest in power, prudence, patience, wisdom, and a deep inner conviction of the need to respect the creation and foster peace. Older people understand the superiority of "being" over "having." (p. 8)

Older people can be living examples of these values.

Related to the concept of mentor is the role of *Beacon of Hope*. For older adults, living hope replaces fleeting wishes. Elders have learned deferred gratification, the ability to postpone pleasure for the sake of long-term satisfaction. They are able to provide a vision of what is yet to be, and a sense of hope. They understand the value of planting now, and reaping later. Reverend Clyde Carleton (1999), Director of Pastoral Care at Oakwood Village in Madison, Wisconsin, shares this story: "I asked an eighty-three year old woman what the greatest thing was that had happened in her life. She said: 'It has not yet happened.' We learn that there may always be a surprise just around the next corner."

Elders can be examples of the fullness of a life of faith. According to Monseigneur Fahey (McDonnell, 1989), "The Gospel message is made credible or incredible to a large extent by older people. If younger churchgoers see older members who are enthusiastic, committed and joyful, their own faith is strengthened and the truth of the Gospel shines through" (p. 31). Founder of the Christian Appalachian Project, Monseigneur Ralph Beiting (1990) describes it this way:

No one can give hope more than one who has walked the road before. Who better than the old can say that sacrifices are worthwhile, that an effort must be made, that the whole journey is worth every step, no matter how painful or unsure. (p. 3)

IMPACT ON CONTEMPORARY SOCIETY

It seems obvious that restoring the role of elder would greatly improve the quality of life for older adults in American culture. But the description of their various roles, past and contemporary, imply that society as whole also has much to gain by rediscovering the importance of elderhood.

Older people represent the "historical memory" of the younger generations. They are the bearers of fundamental human values. Where this memory is lacking, people are rootless, they also lack any capacity to project themselves with hope towards a future that transcends the limits of the present. The family—and hence society as a whole—will benefit from a revaluation of the educational role of older people. (Pontifical Council for the Laity, 1999, p. 11)

It would seem that younger people, particularly children and adolescents, would benefit greatly from the presence of elders in their lives. Pipher (1999) describes the current state of affairs:

A great deal of America's social sickness comes from age segregation. If ten 14 year olds are grouped together, they will form a *Lord of the Flies* culture with its competitiveness and meanness. But if ten people ages 2 to 80 are grouped together, they will fall into a natural age hierarchy that nurtures and teaches them all. For our own mental and societal health, we need to reconnect the age groups. (p. 12)

The need for elder role models was clearly defined in the African culture, as Wimberly (1997) describes:

It was understood that the elders had an important role to play with young people during one of the most difficult times in life, the period between childhood and adulthood. Africans addressed the need of the young during this period to find their identity by guiding them through the rites of passage. Adults, especially elders, were central figures in this process.

The role of elders was to help the young through the transition from youth to adulthood. The elders undertook this role with intentionality. Young people did not become adults by accident or simply by evolution or an unconscious sort of "growing up." (p. 29)

Would elders really make a difference in contemporary society? Would there be less unrest and violence, and more peace, contentment, and harmony? A recent study of the effects of elder mentors on vulnerable youth showed some promising results.

Based on earlier research, it was determined that a variety of interventions have proven successful in helping youth navigate the difficult course through the early teen years. These interventions include:

1. community service activities
2. classroom-based life-skills curriculum
3. parent involvement
4. elder mentors (Taylor and Dryfoos, 1998, p. 44)

In order to study the effects of the elder mentoring, three study groups were established:

1. The program group received all interventions, except mentors.
2. The mentor group received all interventions, including mentors.
3. The control group received no interventions at all. (Taylor and Dryfoos, 1998)

The results indicated that the mentor group scored highest on measures of attitude toward school, attitude toward the future, and attitude toward elders. The mentor group had lower incidents of substance use as well. The research also examined the difference between having highly involved mentors (six hours or more per week) and less involved mentors. It found that youth with highly involved mentors showed better results on a number of measures, including school attendance (Taylor and Dryfoos, 1998).

CONCLUSION

For centuries, in virtually all cultures, older adults had a place of honor in their communities and a valued role as seeker of truth, historian, guide, and teacher of younger people. The work of the elder provided continuity, identity, and integrity to the community, and it gave the elder a sense of purpose in their later years. Today's culture does not hold older people in the same high regard. At best, society has instructed older people to "take it easy and relax" because their work is considered complete. At worst, older people are pushed aside as old fashioned and useless to make way for a newer, modern, and more technologically advanced society.

As a result, communities have suffered a gradual deterioration of their primary values. Society has, in many ways, become disillusioned and has lost hope. It lacks a spiritual core that, in times past, was the domain of elders and the legacy passed on to succeeding generations. Many of today's problems are directly associated with the fact that very important, sacred work is not being done, work that once was done, and only can be done, by elders.

According to Mafico (1997), "Old age was cherished in biblical times because it is a gift denied many. The elders have qualities and attributes that make them indispensable advisers, storytellers, historians, and spiritual leaders in the community" (p. 32). While it may be difficult to solve all of the world's problems, it would be a better place to live for people of all generations if elders were given a place of honor and encouraged to exercise an active role in the community. As Monseigneur Beiting (1990) says: "As I see it, the world needs me more now that I am old than it did when I was young. I sure don't intend to let it down" (p. 1).

REFERENCES

Beiting, R. (1990). From our founder. *The Mountain Spirit* 9(1):1-3.

Bianchi, E. C. (1990). *Aging as a spiritual journey.* New York: Crossroad Publishing Company.

Bly, R. (1990). *Iron John: A book about men.* New York: Vintage Books.

Boucher, T. M. (1991). *Spiritual grandparenting: Bringing our grandchildren to God.* New York: Crossroad Publishing Company.

Campbell, R. A. (1994). *The elders: Seniority within the earliest Christian community.* Edinburgh, Scotland: T & T Clark Ltd.

Carleton, C. (1999). Director of Pastoral Care, Oakwood Lutheran Homes. Personal Correspondence. April 20, 1999.

Cox, F. M. and N. Mberia (1975). *Aging in a changing village society: A Kenyan experience.* International Federation on Aging.

Eschweiler, E. (1999). Retired Pastor. Personal Correspondence. April 18, 1999.

Fahey, C. J. (1987). The third age center. *Pride* 6(3):6-12.

Griffin, R. (1997). Still faithful after all these years. *U.S. Catholic,* 62(10):33-35.

Hagestad, G. O. (1986) Women as kinskeepers. In Pifer, A. and L. Bronte (Eds.), *Our aging society* (pp. 148-158). New York: W.W. Norton and Company.

Mafico, Temba L. J. (1997). Tapping our roots: African and biblical teachings. In Ann S. Wimberly (Ed.), *Honoring African American elders* (pp. 19-33). San Francisco, CA: Jossey-Bass Publishers.

McDonnell, C. (1989). The third age: New challenges for older Catholics. *St. Anthony Messenger* 96(8):29-34.

Palmore, E. (1975). *The honorable elders.* Durham, NC: Duke University Press.

Percy, C. H. (1974). *Growing old in the country of the young.* New York: McGraw-Hill Book Company.

Pipher, M. (1999). The new generation gap. *USA Weekend* March 19-21, p. 12.

Pontifical Council for the Laity (1999). *The dignity of older people and their mission in the Church and in the world.* Vatican City: L'Osservatore Romano, N6-10.

Riley, M. W. and J. Waring (1978). Most of the problems of aging are not biological, but social. In Gross, R., B. Gross, and S. Seidman (Eds.), *The new old: Struggling for decent aging* (pp. 62-70). Garden City, NY: Anchor Books.

Taylor, A. S. and J. G. Dryfoos (1998). Creating a safe passage: Elder mentors and vulnerable youth. *Generations* 22(4):43-48.

Wall, S. (1993). *Wisdom's daughters.* New York: HarperCollins Publishers.

Wilhelm, R. B. (1987). *Grandparents: Advocates, storytellers, and makers of community.* Senior Update Series. Cincinnati, OH: St. Anthony Messenger Press.

Wimberly, A. S. (Ed.) (1997). *Honoring African American elders: A ministry in the soul community.* San Francisco, CA: Jossey-Bass Publishers.

Chapter 3

Spirituality
in Gerontological Theories

David O. Moberg

Theories can influence personal and professional behavior, even when people do not realize that a theory is guiding their actions. For example, competing theories lie behind questions such as whether alcoholism is a disease, the result of an organic chemical imbalance, a consequence of social deprivation, the effect of deliberate acts of the will, or an outcome of spiritually rejecting God. Similarly, when research supported germ theory, it displaced the practice of bloodletting to cure illness.

The word *theory* comes from the Greek *theoria,* a beholding, spectacle, contemplation, or speculation. This means that every theory is a conceptual model that represents a particular way of viewing the world. Its socially constructed meanings direct attention to certain ways of looking at reality while ignoring aspects not covered or considered unimportant by it.

Each theory is a set of logically related statements attempting to explain a class of events. It is tested by testing hypotheses—specific generalizations logically derived from or connected with it, each of which may be verified or rejected through scientific observation. Thus, theories guide research. They are often predictive with statements such as, "If X occurs, Y will also." If Y does not follow X, the hypothesis is rejected.

Theories have practical implications. They can be prescriptive: To obtain a desired result, we act to sustain whatever the theory says is its source or cause. They likewise may be proscriptive: If we do not want a result that damages our interests, such as poverty in old age, we try to prevent or block circumstances the theory posits as its cause.

GERONTOLOGICAL THEORIES

Theories of aging help to organize gerontology as a discipline and to guide geriatric practice in professions like those represented in this book. Theories come from numerous scholarly disciplines (biology, economics, psychology, sociology, etc.). Each is like a philosophical statement about aspects of aging or characteristics of elderly people that separates what its supporters consider important, from details they believe to be irrelevant or nonessential. No theory covers everything. Each enlightens some aspects of the nature of society, social relationships, politics, religion, spirituality, etc., while at the same time ignoring others.

No single theory dominates social gerontology. Some theories compete with one another, but usually it is wise to recognize that they complement one another because each has a different focus of attention. Each sheds a different light on aging, including religion and spirituality. One may apply well to investigations of a given topic, but not well at all to another. The triangulation of applying the perspectives of two or more theories in any given investigation yields far richer results than a dogmatic ideological commitment to one theory alone.

Research may eventually prove the superiority of certain ideological theories, but even then the evaluation of what is superior will rest upon predetermined values, such as beliefs about what is best for human well-being, how best to measure it, and the means for improving it.

SPIRITUALITY AND RELIGION
IN GERONTOLOGICAL THEORY

Spirituality and religion generally have been ignored in theories of aging, but the rapidly expanding evidence of their significance for personal and societal well-being may soon end that neglect.

> Analysis of the reciprocal and interactive relationships of each gerontological theory to spiritual well-being during late life may become one of the most important developments in both qualitative and quantitative research on the role of religion in [physical] health, . . . life satisfaction, psychological health, and holistic well-being. . . . Religion and spirituality infuse all do-

mains of human life, so they should be recognized appropriately in all areas of theoretical and applied gerontology. (Moberg, 1997, pp. 213-214)

The following are a few suggestions toward integrating spirituality and religion into dominant theoretical "schools" of gerontology. Some research evidence supporting each is already available, but it is very scattered. All need further empirical testing, although support for some of them is evident in other chapters of this book.

Disengagement Theory

Disengagement theory (Cumming and Henry, 1961), assumes that both individuals and society benefit when older persons withdraw from roles and activities in which they were previously engaged. Disengagement occurs gradually, is inevitable until death, and is universal. It is mutually satisfying, enhancing the life satisfaction and happiness of withdrawing persons, while helping society maintain equilibrium by fitting younger people into the vacated positions.

Critics of the theory claim it is too simplistic, based upon ethnocentric biases of modern industrial societies, and inconsistent with what often happens when seniors vacate roles. They point to society's loss of the wisdom and experience of aged members and to normative implications that make persons the pawns of society, threatening their freedom and autonomy by mandatory age norms and compulsory retirement laws.

Observational evidence of disengagement policies is not difficult to find in religion, although there is little systematic research on the subject. In many denominations, pastors past the age of fifty are less likely to be called to a congregation with a vacancy than those who are younger. Some congregations seem to have an unwritten rule that members beyond age sixty or seventy, no matter how capable, have served their time, so "new blood" should be appointed or elected to leadership positions. Shut-in members and those in long-term care are often neglected by the "out of sight, out of mind" human tendency.

On the other hand, even when disability or weakness forces discontinued attendance at religious gatherings, people can remain socially engaged if active steps are taken to include them in the spiritual life of their religious community. Mindel and Vaughan (1978) found that over half of the elders aged sixty-two to ninety-eight in their study seemed withdrawn from religion because they did not attend religious services regularly, yet they had high levels of "non-organizational religion"—listening to religious music and services on radio and television, praying, and gaining help for their personal lives from religion, which still was salient in their lives.

Spirituality, however, is another matter. Those who are spiritually alive and alert can continue to grow toward greater spiritual maturity, even when other capabilities are fading. Like the Apostle Paul, they "do not lose heart. Though outwardly we are wasting away, yet inwardly we are being renewed day by day" (2 Corinthians 4:16, NIV). The Duke longitudinal study of aging found that religious attitudes and satisfactions of aging subjects tended to remain much the same over time, but correlations of religious attitudes and activities with happiness, feelings of usefulness, and personal adjustment tended to increase (Blazer and Palmore, 1976).

Activity Theory

The oldest theory in social gerontology is *activity theory,* although it received that name only after, and largely in reaction to, disengagement theory. Some question whether it is a theory at all or only an underlying philosophy or set of ethical standards to guide caregivers of the elderly and leaders of senior groups. As a "golden years" perspective, its emphasis is upon keeping active mentally, physically, and socially as the way to be well adjusted or happy in old age (Havighurst and Albrecht, 1953). Activity offsets the losses experienced by most people during late adulthood. When they retire from work and lose their social identities, people can adapt by comfortable acquiescence (the "rocking chair" of disengagement), but replacement of losses with new activities or consolidation of energy on those that remain is believed to be a more satisfactory adaptation.

Much of the attention given senior adults in religious contexts has focused upon their limitations and losses, burdens and pains. That lopsided approach tends to emphasize what can and should be done *for* them, not ways of serving together *with* them, and even less the ministries that can be provided *by* them. The aging-problems approach tends to impose and strengthen uncomplimentary stereotypes of old age, imparting negative emotions and self-images. It usually fails to call attention to the joys and benefits of old age and retirement. Under its self-fulfilling prophecies, middle-aged people strenuously try to avoid becoming "old" and refuse to tell their age.

Activity theory infuses the ideology of most denominational literature, religious programs for older adults, and educational materials to train the leaders of aging ministries. Their therapeutic goal is to keep older members actively involved in congregational and community life, often with projects and programs designed just for them. Specialized activities can be paced slower, scheduled in the middle of the day, and in other ways allow for differences between elders and younger adults. Older adults are offered opportunities for volunteer services, including prayer chains, "odd-jobs" assistance, friendly visiting, informal counseling, and the encouraging "power of the listening ear." Most volunteers benefit socially, emotionally, and spiritually, even more than do the recipients of their services.

But implementing activity theory can have a downside. Its practical effect is insistence that everybody become or keep busy. Yet that in itself can be a form of tyranny, a dehumanizing *new ageism* (Kalish, 1979) insisting that every older person maintain a lifestyle more appropriate to middle age than to elderhood, with little allowance for different interests and abilities. If one judges "successful aging" only by activities appropriate for middle-aged adults, activity theory can become "little more than a subtle way of glorifying youth at the expense of old age" (Bianchi, 1984, p. 198). That can make many define themselves as worthless failures because they are "slowing down." Might not quietly "inactive" meditating, praying, reading, even selective television viewing, be means for spiritual growth, not simply symptoms of poor adjustment in old age?

Continuity Theory

In reaction to limitations of activity and disengagement theories and stimulated by research evidence, Atchley (1977) formulated *continuity theory*. It assumes that individuals develop habits, preferences, commitments, and other dispositions that become a part of their personalities. As they grow older, "they are predisposed toward maintaining continuity in habits, associations, preferences, and so on. . . . The life-long experience thus creates predispositions that individuals will maintain if at all possible" (p. 27).

People demonstrate *identity continuity* when they continue to see themselves as teachers, railroaders, or members of other occupational roles after retirement. They experience both *internal continuity* when their ideas are persistently structured by memory and *external continuity* when they live in familial environments and interact with familiar people, especially those who knew them at work and retired as part of the same cohort. Continuity does not mean that there is no change, but "simply that change occurs in the *context* of considerable continuity" (Atchley, 1991, p. 104n). Continuity of self and personality, of activities and environments, of relationships, of lifestyle and residence, of roles and activities, and of independence and personal effectiveness is "a central adaptive alternative in coping with many of the changes associated with aging" (p. 260; see also Atchley, 1995).

The best predictor of the religious life of elderly people indeed is their earlier religious orientations. Most retain the same denominational membership or nonmembership as in their middle years, but some deviate from that pattern. Most pastors of evangelical Christian congregations know people who were converted to faith in Jesus Christ during their sixties, seventies, or even older, some from atheism, agnosticism, or non-Christian religions. They also know adults of all ages who are part of the movement from theologically liberal into conservative churches, with fewer moving in the opposite direction.

In addition to externally observable changes by a substantial minority of elderly people, many who retain the same memberships and external religious activities profess to have intensified their faith or deepened their spirituality during later maturity. This usually (but not always) continues a spiritual pilgrimage that began much earlier in life, rather than an abrupt break with adult beliefs and commitments. Brennan and Missinne (1980) asked retrospective questions of a sample of ninety-two independently living senior adults at congregate meal sites and a retirement village. There were no differences between their current and "have you always" responses about belief in God (99 percent), the afterlife (93 percent), and regular church attendance (67 percent); but fewer (59 percent now, 72 percent always) belonged to one or more church-related organizations. On the following three questions, the changes were in the direction of greater spirituality and more feelings of acceptance in their church, despite diminished belonging to its suborganizations:

	Now	Always
Do you consider yourself a religious person?	91%	72%
Do you pray or meditate regularly?	83%	68%
Do you feel accepted by the members of your church?	93%	83%

Continuity theory has been criticized for not sufficiently allowing for external changes in society and for changes of ability and health that modify people's activities, relationships, and self-images. Those (if any) who accept it as an ideology could believe that it is futile to try to help people change engrained worldviews or actions, even those harmful to themselves or others.

The fact that higher percentages of those past age sixty-five than of younger age groups are active church members and more consider religion as very important in their own lives could result from deepened spirituality. Unless this is interpreted as strengthening, deepening, or crystallizing an earlier spiritual orientation, such findings seem to contradict continuity theory (see Chapter 4). However, when the evidence comes only from cross-sectional comparisons of people at different ages, the variations could result from period effects (people reared in the same historical periods are similar to each other), earlier deaths among the less religious people, or other causes (see Moberg, 1997). Perhaps the old proverb applies to spirituality, "What you are now, you are rapidly becoming."

Symbolic Interactionism

A major theoretical school in social psychology is *symbolic interactionism*. Its emphasis is upon the symbolic aspects of relationships that operate during every process of action between persons. For example, whenever two or more people relate to one another, each has his or her own interpretation of what is involved in their relationship, location, and activities. This "definition of the situation" influences what they do and say. Each has an understanding (whether clear or vague) of the roles expected of each person in the group and of one's own self-identity in it. Group members may use laudable or derogatory labels for themselves and others during conversations. Their actions may be patterned or stylized, each acting out expected or unanticipated parts, almost like a scripted drama on the stage.

These are aspects of the processes involved in symbolic interaction, which includes subspecialties like role theory, dramaturgical sociology, socialization analysis, labeling theory, and in some respects, ethnomethodology, phenomenology, and existentialism. What goes on in the mind via language, communication, and thinking, spills over into interpretations of meanings, personal and group identities, and required or expected behavior, all intermingled in ever-changing processes and actions within, between, and among people.

Aging is a dynamic process revolving around interaction between persons and others in their social world whose interpretations of and reactions to physiological and incidental changes greatly influence what happens to each aging individual. The values held by groups to which persons belong help to determine the manner and extent to which disengagement, activity, or continuity predominates. That certainly applies in regard to religion and even spirituality. Religious roles and their enactment structure people's perceptions, influence their motivations, and shape their identities and meanings in life (see Holm, 1995).

Positive and negative stereotypes of older people, definitions of who is "old," and interpretations of the roles removed from, offered to, or imposed upon elders in religious contexts greatly influence their self-concepts, activities, mental health, and expectations for the future. These have a profound impact upon their self-esteem, sense of relative deprivation or appreciation compared to other people, withdrawal from or entry into specific groups (religious or other), and self-fulfilling prophecies about the "senility" or wisdom of elders.

Theologically, all people, young and old, capable and disabled, whatever their ethnicity or race, are equal in most religious groups. The Bible insists that all people are created in the image of God, but also that everybody has sinned and fallen short of that glory. Yet all can be redeemed as a free gift of God's grace through the redemption that is freely offered to everyone through Jesus Christ, so they can be restored to the dignity of spiritual membership in God's family. The symbolic interactive impact of this may help explain why more elderly people are members of churches than of all other social organizations put together.

What happens in religious groups thus has a profound impact upon what happens in the minds and behavior of members. Life satisfaction, anticipatory socialization for the afterlife stage of existence, and high or low levels of spirituality, are influenced by and sometimes products of the patterns of symbolic interaction in worship services, pastoral care, small groups such as Bible studies and prayer circles, stylized interchanges such as friendly visiting for a church or synagogue, and casual communications with as few as one other member. Unfortunately, some religious congregations still unintentionally sustain ageism, exclude young and old handicapped persons, and in other ways make participation impossible or uncomfortable (see Moberg, 1982; Thornburgh, 1994).

Exchange Theory

The exchange of services and goods is a central topic of economics, but exchange is even broader in gerontological theory. It assumes that people act to maximize material and nonmaterial rewards and benefits and to minimize the costs of losing them. *Exchange theory* views social life as a series of exchanges that add to or subtract from one's power, prestige, and possessions. Social goods include psychological satisfaction, need gratification, and experiential pleasure besides economic and material possessions.

In its early development, Martin (1971) used exchange theory to help understand power relationships in visiting patterns among family members. Elderly persons with resources such as financial wealth and interesting stories to tell may put their relatives in a dependent position, while elders with little power outside of family obligations may have difficulty motivating visits and pay a high sociopsychological price for them.

While exploring why social interaction and activity often decrease in old age, Dowd (1975) concluded that exchange relationships were a better explanation than disengagement and activity theory. The power advantage has shifted from elders to society via mandatory retirement in exchange for pensions, Social Security, and Medicare, producing imbalanced relationships to their disadvantage. The norm of reciprocity, emphasized especially by anthropologists, calls for equivalent payments when goods or deeds of service are received, so the young-old are encouraged to remain productive wage earners. But groups such as children, mentally or physically handicapped persons, and the elderly are unable to repay their helpers, so a norm of beneficence, including government services for the old-old who are not expected to repay, calls into play nonrational sentiments like love, loyalty, duty to parents, and gratitude for past contributions.

Infirm persons can make significant exchange contributions via their spirituality. Long after physical strength has waned or disabilities intruded to make them incapable of giving physically demanding services like running errands or providing child care for family members, elderly believers can serve others by simply giving encouragement and counsel. They can listen to others' tales of joy or grief, share experience-based insights and perspectives upon others' burdens, remind them of Scriptural counsel that meets their needs, share interesting vignettes from their own life story, help them to see "the silver lining" of the "dark clouds" of life, bring their knowledge and skills to bear upon problems that need solution, and pray that God will satisfy them. Those who are bedridden give others the opportunity to serve, which in itself can be rewarding, whether seen from an exchange or other symbolic interaction perspective. As Jesus said, "It is more blessed [rewarding, satisfaction providing] to give than to receive" (Acts 20:35, NIV).

Ministries with and for the aging can be interpreted from the perspective of long-range exchanges in which past generations who once provided goods and services, including church buildings, equipment, and duties performed in religious offices and committees, are now receiving deferred rewards, while the younger generation is building its "social credit" toward the time when they themselves will need to collect benefits.

Those ministries also can be viewed as fulfilling biblical teachings to love one's neighbor as oneself, to provide for widows and the poor, and to serve God and others faithfully with whatever spiritual gifts one has been given (Romans 12:4-8; 1 Corinthians 12:4-31). The belief that people can exchange goodness on earth for eternal salvation is very common in some Christian and other groups, but the Bible boldly states that such is impossible (see Ephesians 2:8-10; Titus 3:4-8). Yet believers who please God will be rewarded (2 Corinthians 5:9-10).

Stage Theories

Obviously, people go through various stages of life. This is reflected in religious education classes that meet the different needs, interests, and levels of intellectual and social development by groups of babies in the nursery, children at preschool to junior and intermediate levels, high school and college-aged youth, young adults, and other adult groups up to the retirement years.

Some *stage theories* differentiate levels of adult development. Perhaps most prominent is Erikson's (1963, 1982) psychoanalytic theory with eight stages based upon complex interactions of societal values and psychological growth. Each stage has a developmental task to accomplish for normal personality development before going on to the next. In early adulthood, e.g., the emphasis is upon *intimacy,* especially with a friend or mate, uniting or merging one's personal identity with that of another. The failure to do so is *isolation.* By middle adulthood the emphasis is upon *generativity,* the ability to support others and contribute to one's social world. Those who fail experience *stagnation.* In later life the main issue is *ego integrity,* the ability to see one's life as having been meaningful and to accept oneself as worthwhile, in contrast to the *despair* of self- and life-rejection that inclines one toward depression and fear of death. What occurs spiritually at each stage influences all future stages. Although difficult to use in research, Erikson's theory has considerably influenced additional theorizing, clinical psychology, and some theological studies of human development (e.g., Loder, 1998).

Fowler's Stages of Faith

Building upon personality theory and Kohlberg's (1969, 1981) work on stages of moral judgment, Fowler (1981, 1991) theorized that faith development is a sequence of six stages in which individuals cognitively and emotionally shape their relationship to a transcendent center(s) of value:

1. *Intuitive-projective faith* (ages two through seven) when a child becomes aware of self and God
2. *Mythic-literal faith* (ages seven through twelve) when family-specified perspectives and meanings of morals and God are internalized
3. *Synthetic-conventional faith* (adolescence onward) when faith is accepted without critical examination and group norms are sustained

4. *Individuative-reflective faith* (early to mid-twenties or beyond) when ideological faith is critically examined and one's own belief system reconstructed
5. *Conjunctive faith* (midlife and beyond) when disillusionment with that belief system sets in and one is caught between it and openness to other religious traditions
6. *Universalizing faith* (late life) that brings oneness with the power of being or divinity, willingness to promote justice in the world, and fellowship with others regardless of their faith stage or religious tradition

Many people stop developing at the third stage, and few, if any, attain the sixth level, the allegedly highest degree of spiritual maturation.

Fowler's theory has influenced much religious education (Dykstra and Parks, 1986), but it is based upon the value assumptions of theological liberalism, universalism, and relativism. It relies more heavily upon the intellectual and cognitive aspects of development than upon its emotional and motivational aspects. Loder (1998) says the stages illuminate "stages of ego and the capacity of ego to construct meaning. But they are not stages of faith in any biblical or theological sense" (p. 255). In addition, Fowler's normative goal of universalizing contains the seeds of falsification for his own theory. "What kind of a model is it that sets up a normative goal that, if it is attained, would expose the model itself to be inadequate and in error?" (Loder, 1998, p. 258). The theory not only fails to provide an adequate picture of "faithing" as a whole, but by emphasis upon the *form* of thinking rather than its precise *content,* it deletes much that is important to persons who are developing (Loder, 1998, p. 259).

Koenig's (1994, pp. 87-104) critique of Fowler's theory, emerging from his psychiatric expertise and research on religion and aging, draws attention to many aspects that may require reformulation. He especially questions the wisdom of applying a cognitively based model to measure faith development in older adults, many of whom have limited education, chronic physical illness, and/or cognitive dysfunction.

> The opportunity to advance in faith, rather than being procurable only by a select few, should be available even to a small child, a retarded adult, or an elderly person with a stroke or slowly advancing organic brain syndrome. . . . [T]hese stages represent an intellectualized version of faith that may not be relevant for the

uneducated, cognitively impaired, or psychologically unsophisticated. (Koenig, 1994, pp. 97, 103)

Koenig therefore built his own theory of *religious faith development,* giving major attention to biblically based faith content. He emphasizes the triune nature of humanity with interacting parts of body (physical), mind (psychosocial), and spirit (soul—the supernatural, relatively constant part that endures after bodily death). Faith is believing, experiencing, and acting, not belief alone. "Religious faith development is a process during which persons' relationship with God (or Jesus, for the Christian) becomes their ultimate concern and primary motivation in life" (Koenig, 1994, p. 113). Each person follows a unique path of faith development, moving both forward and backward throughout the life span. Mature faith is manifested differently by children, young and old adults, intellectually gifted persons, and the cognitively impaired. It is described and expressed differently by the members of different religious traditions, even those within Christianity. Born out of adversity and applied through loving actions, mature faith "may act as a source of strength, peace, and hope for persons in later life as they face the trials of aging. . . . Even with advancing cognitive impairment, the ability to participate in relationship with God is one of the last human capacities to be lost before consciousness itself ceases" (pp. 133-134). The capacity to trust (to believe and have faith) is the first psychosocial task learned by the growing infant and one of the last to depart as life ends (p. 508).

Theological orientations, personal experiences, and presuppositions of theorists influence the process and content of developmental stage theories of spirituality. They are easier to illustrate than to test empirically, so preexisting values influence their acceptance or rejection by others. For example, many evangelical Christians believe Fowler's theory contradicts their Bible-based belief that there is only one way to God and salvation—faith in Jesus Christ (John 14:6; Acts 4:12; etc.). Their emphasis is upon biblical teachings, including that the transformation from spiritual death to spiritual life through faith in Jesus Christ should be followed by growth and development. They realize that one can get stuck at a worldly or carnal level of spiritual infancy (1 Corinthians 3:1-3) instead of growth toward the spiritual maturity of "attaining to the whole measure of the fullness of Christ" (Ephesians 4:13, NIV). Like Koenig, they give primary attention to the content of faith—in what do people put their trust?—while Fowler focuses more upon its structure.

Conclusion

The many theories on stages of religious development (see also Moody and Carroll, 1997) differ in their points of departure and their philosophical and theological foundations. The empirical evidence on them is not yet solid and sometimes yields contradictory results. "There is no 'United Grand Theory' of . . . religious development" (Tamminen and Nurmi, 1995, p. 302). Pragmatically most important is the fact that spiritual growth is possible long after other forms of growth are past. However it changes, spirituality is a domain of humanity in which the quest for wholeness and holiness is a lifelong developmental task.

Stratification and Subculture Theories

Closely related to stage theories are those that emphasize how social life is organized by age categories (e.g., Riley, Johnson, and Foner, 1972). *Age stratification theories* typically give attention to structured inequalities related to age, with one-way transitions from young to next older. Age-graded roles, such as compulsory retirement rules for clergy, still found in many religious groups have built-in definitions that are independent of the specific persons who occupy them. People who are part of a given cohort tend to flow through these stages of life under social pressures to live in ways viewed as appropriate for their age. Popular discussions of the generation gap between youth, their parental generation, and grandparents reflect this.

The concept of an *aging subculture* overlaps with stratification and stage theories. Rose (1965) believed that the growing number of aging people in the population and the improved means of interaction among them are causing formation of a subgroup with distinct ideas, values, beliefs, behaviors, and preferences. Ageism excludes older people from participation in major sectors of society and enhances their consciousness of common interests. It pushes them toward formation of aging ghettoes like retirement communities and neighborhoods in cities and small towns and the founding of new organizations such as the Gray Panthers and the AARP (American Association of Retired Persons). This results in an aging self-concept, group pride, and a political "gray lobby."

There are golden-age clubs, senior centers, and other subgroups for senior citizens in many religious congregations, and clear evidence suggests that the population past age sixty-five is on the whole more religious than younger age cohorts. The formation of organizations for elders focused around religious interests, like the Christian Association of PrimeTimers, further reflects the subcultural perspective. Nevertheless, the elderly remain divided in numerous ways, including their levels of poverty and wealth, political loyalties, and religion, so a solid senior bloc has not yet emerged.

Conflict Theory

The main focus of *conflict theory* is upon structured inequality among subgroups in society. It holds that conflict (including rivalry, competition, etc.) and value dissensus (lack of agreement) are normal in society, if not its basic social process. Persons and groups are continually struggling to obtain scarce resources and powerful groups exploit the weak.

One version is *Social Darwinism,* which holds that society evolves by survival of the fittest, so there should be no controls on competition. Ageism results as industrialization and modernization shift the elderly from an advantaged position of being the source of wisdom in society to uselessness in production. Negative stereotypes, false conceptions of the worth of elders, and costs of supporting people no longer in the labor force presumably divide workers from retirees, disuniting the working class and sustaining the power of the wealthy. The drive toward legalizing euthanasia reflects this theory.

Marxism emphasizes exploitation of the working class (proletariats) by the bourgeoisie. Those who hold power and property in society control politics, education, the mass media, and religion. As "the opiate of the people," religion is a tool of the power structure that makes the masses content to stay in their place. It gives the poor and the elderly comfort with hope of "pie in the sky by and by," an expression many Marxist have used for a better life beyond the grave. Governmental control of religion in the People's Republic of China, where only the Three-Self Church is legal, centuries of state churches in Europe, and governmentally supported Islam are examples of the control of religion by political power structures.

Conflicts within and between denominations, "church fights" in congregations and parishes, and political struggles that have a religious base or use religious groups to advance their goals also illustrate conflict theory. They influence spirituality even though they fit more clearly in the category of religion. Theological struggles often are more clearly centered around spiritual issues, as in the conflicts between good and evil, God and Satan, and the spirit and the flesh.

Contrasting sociological theories centered around cooperation and beneficence to either complement or stand in contrast to conflict theories are not formally developed in gerontology.

CONCLUSIONS

The theories presented here are complementary ways of looking at aging, not alternatives from which to choose. Each provides a different perspective on the social context and psychological processes of aging. Many additional theoretical orientations in gerontology (e.g., Matras, 1990, pp. 197-229), psychology, sociology, and related disciplines can be applied to the study of spirituality and religion, so we have only skimmed the surface. Lanum and Birren (1995) have summarized theories of aging based upon biological, psychological, and social determinism and spelled out their ecological theory counterpart. Hood's (1995) handbook on religious experience has chapters on depth psychologies and on developmental, cognitive, affective, behavioral, attribution, attachment, and transpersonal theories, as well as on six faith traditions.

Even genetic and biochemical theories have potential value for in-depth studies of spirituality in aging. There is substantial evidence to support the theory of *nonreductive physicalism,* which holds that "statements about the physical nature of human beings made from the perspective of biology or neuroscience are about exactly the same entity as statements made about the spiritual nature of persons from the point of view of theology or religious traditions" (Brown, Murphy, and Malony, 1998, p. xiii).

The theories discussed in this chapter were developed in the context of American society. Their applications to religion and spirituality most clearly fit people with a Christian religious heritage. In many other cultures, aging roles, philosophies, and interpretations of spirituality are considerably different. For example, the religious and cultural literature of India presents many images of aging, seen as a marker of the journey of life, as growth and development toward maturity, as decline and loss, and as an accomplice of death. Sociocultural and spiritual values are commingled, and all of life is interpreted in terms of four stages: the student, married life, withdrawal from the family, and complete renunciation during old age when many men engage in ascetic pilgrimages, scriptural studies, or other spiritual activities (Tilak, 1989).

Amidst the broad diversity of Hinduism, transcendence of the spiritual over the profane takes precedence over doctrinal concerns with an emphasis on disciplines and techniques that are relatively independent of theology (Puhakka, 1995; see Raman, 1998). Buddhism is possibly even more diverse and complex (Hong, 1995; Chit, 1988). As theistic religions, Judaism (Jacobs, 1995; Olitzky and Borowitz, 1995) and Islam (Moughrabi, 1995) are closer to Christianity, yet characterized by a medley of spiritual and religious perspectives.

Obviously, gerontological theories of spirituality are greatly underdeveloped. They are a rich potential domain for scholars and researchers to develop and test.

REFERENCES

Atchley, Robert C. (1977). *The social forces in later life,* Second edition. Belmont, CA: Wadsworth.

Atchley, Robert C. (1991). *Social forces and aging: An introduction to social gerontology,* Sixth editon. Belmont, CA: Wadsworth.

Atchley, Robert C. (1995). The continuity of the spiritual self. In Kimble, Melvin A., Susan H. McFadden, James W. Ellor, and James J. Seeber (Eds.), *Aging, spirituality, and religion: A handbook* (pp. 68-73). Minneapolis, MN: Fortress Press.

Bianchi, Eugene C. (1984). *Aging as a spiritual journey.* New York: Crossroad Publishing Co.

Blazer, Daniel and E. Palmore (1976). Religion and aging in a longitudinal panel. *The Gerontologist* 16(1):82-85.

Brennan, Constance L. and Leo E. Missinne (1980). Personal and institutionalized religiosity of the elderly. In Thorson, James A. and Thomas C. Cook Jr. (Eds.), *Spiritual well-being of the elderly* (pp. 92-99). Springfield, IL: Charles C Thomas.

Brown, Warren S., Nancey Murphy, and H. Newton Malony (Eds.). (1998). *Whatever happened to the soul?: Scientific and theological portraits of human nature.* Minneapolis, MN: Fortress Press.

Chit, Daw Khin Myo (1988). Add life to years the Buddhist way. In Clements, William M. (Ed.), *Religion, aging and health: A global perspective* (pp. 39-67). Binghamton, NY: The Haworth Press.

Cumming, Elaine and W. E. Henry (1961). *Growing old: The process of disengagement.* New York: Basic Books.

Dowd, James J. (1975). Aging as exchange: A preface to theory. *Journal of Gerontology* 30(5):584-594.

Dykstra, Craig and Sharon Parks (1986). *Faith development and Fowler.* Birmingham, AL: Religious Education Press.

Erikson, Erik H. (1963). *Childhood and society,* Second edition. New York: Norton.

Erikson, Erik H. (1982). *The life cycle completed.* New York: Norton.

Fowler, James W. (1981). *Stages of faith: The psychology of human development and the quest for meaning.* San Francisco: Harper & Row.

Fowler, James W. (1991). *Weaving the new creation: Stages of faith and the public church.* San Francisco: Harper & Row.

Havighurst, Robert and Ruth Albrecht (1953). *Older people.* New York: Longmans, Green.

Holm, Nils G. (1995). Role theory and religious experience. In Hood, Ralph W. Jr. (Ed.), *Handbook of religious experience* (pp. 397-420). Birmingham, AL: Religious Education Press.

Hong, Gui-Young (1995). "Buddhism and Religious Experience." In Hood, Ralph W. Jr. (Ed.), *Handbook of Religious Experience* (pp. 87-121). Birmingham, AL: Religious Education Press.

Hood, Ralph W. Jr. (Ed.) (1995). *Handbook of religious experience.* Birmingham, AL: Religious Education Press.

Jacobs, Janet L. (1995). Judaism and religious experience. In Hood, Ralph W. Jr. (Ed.), *Handbook of Religious Experience* (pp. 13-29). Birmingham, AL: Religious Education Press.

Kalish, Richard A. (1979). The new ageism and the failure models: A polemic. *The Gerontologist* 19(4):398-402.

Koenig, Harold G. (1994). *Aging and God: Spiritual pathways to mental health in midlife and later years.* Binghamton, NY: The Haworth Press.

Kohlberg, Lawrence (1969). Stage and sequence: The cognitive-developmental approach to socialization. In Goslin, D. (Ed.), *Handbook of socialization theory and research* (pp. 347-480). New York: Rand McNally.

Kohlberg, Lawrence (1981). *The philosophy of moral development.* San Francisco: HarperCollins.

Lanum, Jackie C. and James E. Birren (1995). Adult development theories and concepts. In Kimble, Melvin A., Susan H. McFadden, James W. Ellor, and James J. Seeber (Eds.), *Aging, spirituality, and religion: A handbook* (pp. 511-532). Minneapolis, MN: Fortress Press.

Loder, James E. (1998). *The logic of the spirit: Human development in theological perspective.* San Francisco: Jossey-Bass Publishers.

Martin, J. David (1971). Power, dependence, and the complaints of the elderly: A social exchange perspective. *Aging and Human Development* 2(2):108-112.

Matras, Judah (1990). *Dependency, obligations, and entitlements: A new sociology of aging, the life course, and the elderly.* Englewood Cliffs, NJ: Prentice-Hall.

Mindel, Charles H. and C. Edwin Vaughan (1978). A multidimensional approach to religiosity and disengagement. *Journal of Gerontology* 33(1):103-108.

Moberg, David O. (1982). Is your church an honest ally or a friendly foe of the aged? *Journal of Christian Education* 3(1):51-64.

Moberg, David O. (1997). Religion and aging. In Ferraro, Kenneth F. (Ed.), *Gerontology: Perspectives and issues* (pp. 193-220). New York: Springer Publishing Co.

Moody, Harry R. and David Carroll (1997). *The five stages of the soul: Charting the spiritual passages that shape our lives.* New York: Anchor/Doubleday.

Moughrabi, Fouad (1995). Islam and religious experience. In Hood, Ralph W. Jr. (Ed.), *Handbook of religious experience* (pp. 72-86). Birmingham, AL: Religious Education Press.

NIV: *The Holy Bible,* New International Version (1984). Colorado Springs, CO: International Bible Society.

Olitzky, Kerry M. and Eugene B. Borowitz (1995). A Jewish perspective. In Kimble, Melvin A., Susan H. McFadden, James W. Ellor, and James J. Seeber (Eds.), *Aging, spirituality, and religion: A handbook* (pp. 389-402). Minneapolis, MN: Fortress Press.

Puhakka, Kaisa (1995). Hinduism and religious experience. In Hood, Ralph W. Jr. (Ed.), *Handbook of religious experience* (pp. 122-143). Birmingham, AL: Religious Education Press.

Raman, V. V. (1998). A Hindu view on science and spirituality. *Science & Spirit* 9(5, December):6-7.

Riley, Matilda W., M. Johnson, and Anne Foner (1972). *Aging and society, Volume 3: A sociology of age stratification.* New York: Russell Sage Foundation.

Rose, Arnold M. (1965). The subculture of the aging: A framework for research in social gerontology. In Rose, Arnold M. and Warren A Peterson (Eds.), *Older people and their social world* (pp. 3-16). Philadelphia: F. A. Davis Co.

Tamminen, Kalevi and Kari E. Nurmi (1995). Developmental theories and religious experience. In Hood, Ralph W. Jr. (Ed.), *Handbook of religious experience* (pp. 269-311). Birmingham, AL: Religious Education Press.

Thornburgh, Ginny (Ed.) (1994). *That all may worship: An interfaith welcome to people with disabilities.* Washington, DC: National Organization on Disability.

Tilak, Shrinivas (1989). *Religion and aging in the Indian tradition.* Albany, NY: State University of New York Press.

RESEARCH AND SPIRITUALITY

The use of scientific methods to investigate spirituality is a relatively recent innovation. Spirituality is so ineffable, transcendent, and sacred that investigating it seems to some impossible and to some, deceptive or sinful. Nevertheless, as dicussed in Chapter 1, many other "unobservable" subjects have become respected topics for investigation in the social and behavioral sciences.

In this section, we shall survey some of the reasons why research on spirituality is important and some commonly used, but defective, ways to do it. Then we shall present a better approach, the use of modern research methods, together with examples of rich findings that already have accumulated from their application to religiousness and spirituality. Next we survey some attitudes toward death and dying that have been brought to awareness through qualitative research and, finally, the findings of a study of age differences in spirituality among women attending a Christian retreat.

Chapter 4

Research on Spirituality

David O. Moberg

This chapter addresses the importance and feasibility of research on spirituality, prescientific interests in such work, and representative findings from investigations of the subject.

People who accept the Bible as a divine guide to faith, conduct, and spirituality rightly argue that only God is the ultimate and fully righteous judge, hence evaluator, of any person's spirituality. Some of them conclude, therefore, that human evaluation is sinful. Yet the Bible includes many prescientific commands and instructions to God's people to engage in evaluation (e.g., Numbers 13; Psalm 34:8; Proverbs 24:3-6; Jeremiah 6:27; Lamentations 3:40; 2 Corinthians 13:5; Galatians 6:4; 1 Thessalonians 5:21-22; Romans 12:2). That is done best today with the help of scientific and scholarly methodologies (see Moberg, 1999). But beyond the goal of expanding academic knowledge, is there any good reason to do research on spirituality?

WHY IS RESEARCH ON SPIRITUALITY IMPORTANT?

Most, if not all, religious groups want to enhance their members' spirituality. Some apply time-honored traditions as the basis for their methods to accomplish that goal. Others rely on recent educational or psychological philosophies. Many attempt to fit contemporary social contexts by reinterpreting scriptural principles. Because each actually accomplishes its spiritual goals for those persons who become the visible core of its membership, leaders tend to assume that they are doing what is right for everyone. But is it not possible that whatever serves, helps, and attracts a few people might also alienate and harm many others? And may not those who are helped be aided even more if the methods and techniques of service delivery were modified? Research can help to find the answers.

Accountability to demonstrate the worth of programs and services is ever more important in our complex, urbanized, and usually impersonal society. Federal and state agencies, including Medicare and Medicaid, insist upon compliance with laws and regulations to protect clients, staff members, and society at large. Cost accounting has become a major issue in the health industry and other professions that are driven as much by the economic crunch as by concern for human well-being.

The importance of spirituality to the overall well-being of people, whether it is labeled as an aspect of life satisfaction, health, shalom, total wellness, or something else, is increasingly recognized. As a result, pressures to bring it and its various components into the domain of evaluation and measurement are mounting (Moberg, 1979). As attention to spirituality grows, the human services to enhance it, especially those provided by nonreligious sponsors, are in danger of being evaluated more by economics than by their less tangible contributions to wholistic well-being.

Examples of Researchable Issues

Thousands of significant questions about the value of attention to spirituality in the various caring professions can be addressed through social, economic, psychological, and epidemiological research. The following are a few examples.

Chaplains in hospitals, nursing homes, prisons, the military, retirement communities, etc., are under pressure to demonstrate that their services are worthwhile. Do they really help hospital patients feel better despite their disabilities? Do they help people recover more rapidly from illness? Do they improve the morale and efficiency of military personnel, contribute to the rehabilitation of prisoners, and reduce the recidivism of exoffenders? Often the most significant administrative question is whether a chaplaincy can prove its worth by reducing overall costs.

The spiritual component in nursing is increasingly recognized (see Shelly and Fish, 1988; Carson, 1989). Spiritual care that complements conventional therapy promotes healing, relieves patients' discomfort and pain, reduces the need for medication, alleviates spiritual distress, etc. But it arguably takes extra staff time and thus increases the expenses of patient care. Is it a worthwhile contributor to the humanitarian goals of health care? Does it pay for itself in terms of the financial bottom line?

Should physicians and surgeons be concerned with the whole person, rather than only with their patients' presenting ailments or problematic body parts? Is there a payoff that compensates financially or by improved recovery for the extra time needed to pay attention to spirituality?

Many spiritual directors, counselors, clinicians, and chaplains think they deserve to receive financial support from health insurance, Medicare, Medicaid, and fees for services. Does research show that their services are fiscally viable?

Does research prove that spirituality does or does not belong in the educational curricula and training programs of social workers and other human service professionals?

Should the budgets of church congregations and synagogues include funds for a psychological clinic, parish nurse, or disability ministry?

What are the unplanned and unintended results of religious activities designed to improve the spiritual wellness of participants?

Do these and other spiritual services really pay for themselves? Do they improve life satisfaction, directly or indirectly? Or do they increase human misery by putting a load of guilt, fear, and worry into the minds of those whom they allegedly serve?

Good research can help to answer these and other significant questions. Often it will satisfy the needs of agency administrators and other staff persons, while also informing skeptical care providers, donors to charitable organizations, taxpayers, and the insurers, legislators, and others who control purse strings.

CASUAL EVALUATIONS AND ASSESSMENTS

Evaluations of spirituality services often take the form of stories about persons or incidents that illustrate the worth or worthlessness that the narrator wishes to emphasize. Anecdotes indeed are an important component of any serious effort to study the entire picture, but case studies can be chosen to fit the purposes of the narrator. Hence they often are judged critically as probable exceptions, unique instances that are noteworthy just because they represent unusual rather than normal results of whatever service or program is under consideration. Humanity is so diverse that there nearly always are "outliers," exceptions to the pattern that is typical of most people in similar circumstances.

Possibly the most common form of evaluation is the sharing of opinions. Sometimes this is done relatively democratically, listening systematically to all sides of debates. More often, however, some people's opinions carry more weight than others' in the decision-making process. Regardless, all opinions tend to be biased by self-interests, value commitments, ideologies, traditions, educational philosophies, organizational memberships, and the like. A high degree of consensus among staff members does not necessarily produce fairness and objectivity on whatever question is under consideration because the same biases may have governed their recruitment and retention. They are likely to notice especially the desirable effects of the programs and services they have established, while critics notice mostly those that are undesirable. Neither side is predisposed to see the entire picture.

Committees to deal with local issues of religious congregations often are equivalent to research teams. However, they are tempted to notice, gather, and report only the facts that support conclusions they have already reached and to ignore or rationalize away any evidence unfavorable to those prejudgments. Such cardstacking is a violation of good research methodology. It is one form of dishonesty or lying, even when done with good intentions.

Because of these and other limitations of casual evaluations of the consequences of services to enhance spirituality, it is advisable to gather objective evidence through systematic research. Good research helps to answer administrative and professional questions. Is the program doing both good and harm? What are its mistakes and shortcomings? How can we improve the good that is accomplished? How can mistakes be eliminated or corrected?

RESEARCH FINDINGS

Basically the same procedural principles (see Chapter 15) relate to both scientific studies in the social, behavioral, epidemiological, and other disciplines that test hypotheses and develop theories to expand basic knowledge and to applied evaluations of the effectiveness and efficiency of specific programs and activities that aim to improve their service delivery. There already are many research tools for studying religion. Nine of the 126 indexes and scales described by Hill and Hood (1999) include the word *spiritual* in their titles, but many others pertain to spirituality as well as religiousness.

Numerous research questions related to spirituality have been answered, at least partly or provisionally. This section summarizes only a few examples of discoveries already made. Some are firmly established by replications; others are preliminary and tentative. All deserve additional investigation to determine whether the findings apply to all people or only to certain ethnic, cultural, or religious groups.

Scientific and scholarly investigations are expanding so rapidly that keeping up with all of the work on religion and spirituality could be one's full-time occupation. Therefore the following sections summarize only a few highlights of findings to date. Details of the reports are found in the references cited, which also lead to hundreds of other studies widely scattered in the literature of many disciplines and professions. Readers who desire an in-depth understanding or who wish to critique the research should use the original reports to determine the strengths and weaknesses of each study, to identify missing or unfinished investigations it suggests, and to discover its implications for action.

Age Differences in Spirituality

With few exceptions, research on numerous groups of Americans has shown that the levels of religious beliefs, behavior, and experiences that reflect spirituality increase with age (Koenig, 1995b, pp. 3-29; Moberg, 1997). Despite racial, religious, and cultural variations, the main exception is diminished attendance at religious services among the old-old who have problems of health and mobility. Their reduced participation in organizational religiosity, however, is often accompanied by high levels of nonorganizational religiosity—praying, listening to religious radio programs and music, watching religious television, and gaining help from religion to understand their own lives (Mindel and Vaughan, 1978). This raises questions about continuity theory, which may apply to most individuals only when crude measures are used.

A common explanation of age differences half a century ago was that age variations represent a cohort difference, each younger generation being less religious as secularization sweeps through society. However, the same age pattern has been repeated again and again in succeeding generations, so the best current explanation is that the aging process itself, rather than a cohort or period effect, explains the deepened spirituality of late life.

The differential survival hypothesis holds that persons who are more spiritual and religiously committed have lifestyles that reduce their mortality. They are less likely than others to use tobacco, abuse alcohol and drugs, engage in premarital sex and adultery, become divorced, and have habits harmful to health. They are more likely to belong to supportive social networks and to experience serenity and peace with other people, themselves, and God. Their lower age-specific mortality rates throughout adulthood could be a significant source of the higher average spirituality in each older generation (Moberg, 1997). A study of over 20,000 U.S. adults estimates that religious involvement prolongs life by about seven years (Hummer et al., 1999).

There is also evidence of actual changes in the religiousness of persons with age (see Chapter 6). Ellor's (1997) analysis of data from 148 participants in preconferences for the White House Conference on Aging found that 86 percent had a different perception of God from that of their childhood, and 74 percent felt closer to God. Other changes pertained to more prayer (61 percent), more application of their faith in daily life (59 percent), and a deeper sense of spirituality (61 percent).

Duke University studies found that most hospitalized patients say their religion became more important to them as they grew older (only 5 percent say its importance decreased), so Koenig (1997, pp. 44-46) noted that evidence is mounting that aging itself affects the interest in religion. "Existential concerns at this time in life might prompt aging persons to reexamine their views about God or perhaps adopt a religious worldview to help cope with stress and life change" (p. 45).

Spirituality and Physical Health

Hundreds of publications have reported research on the effects of religion and spirituality on health. In his extensive bibligraphic study Koenig (1995b) concluded that, in spite of a most ardent search for contrary evidence, "Most studies reported here have found a positive relationship between religious beliefs, behaviors, and mental or physical health" (p. xv). For example, various studies have revealed an inverse relationship between religious commitment and hypertension, and strongly committed persons have significantly lower blood pressure, fewer strokes, better health, and less pain from cancer and other illness or surgery than similar persons with low religious commitment (Koenig, 1995b; see also Koenig, 1997, and Koenig, Smiley, and Gonzales, 1988). Both religious affiliation and regular attendance at religious services appear to buffer the need for and length of hospitalization (Koenig and Larson, 1998).

Despite methodological limitations and heterogeneity in religious measures, these findings point consistently, though not quite unanimously, to a positive health promoting role for religion. Still, many social scientists and biomedical researchers maintain "a sort of 'collective amnesia' . . . that serves to blot out these data or to downplay their significance" (Levin, 1994, p. xvi). They, along with gerontologists in general, have been "colossally blind to the religious dimension of human aging" (Moody, 1994, p. x).

Neglecting these findings results in part from efforts to impose naturalistic interpretations upon them. In addition, clinical practitioners who treat disturbed persons sometimes see some of the worst aspects of religion. Besides, as with nearly everything connected with humanity, there are exceptions to the general pattern. Psychologists Richards and Bergin (1997, pp. 86-88) nevertheless conclude that none of the natural explanations of religion's beneficial power would endure without invoking the influence of God and that this is consistent with Levin's (1995) notion of a superempirical healing energy that is activated by religion.

Prayer

The most frequent form of invoking God in most Christian circles is asking for healing of illness and recovery from surgery. "Prayer changes things" is a common motto in believers' homes, although "God changes things when people pray" seems closer to scriptural teachings. Therapists, however, have tended to see prayer as only a psychological boost or cathartic release for those who pray rather than an external means for actual healing.

A significant experiment to test the effectiveness of intercessory prayer was conducted at San Francisco General Hospital (Byrd, 1988). All patients admitted to its coronary care unit during a nine-month period were invited to become part of a prospective double-blind study. The 393 who gave informed consent (only fifty-seven refused) were assigned randomly by computer to receive (experimental group) or not receive (controls) the prayers of "born again" Catholic and Protestant Christians over and above their normal hospital treatment. Neither the patients, staff, physicians, or project director knew who was in each group. Each experimental patient was randomly assigned to from three to seven intercessors who were given the patient's first name, diagnosis, general condition, and pertinent updates. Intercessors prayed daily until discharge from the hospital for survival, rapid recovery, prevention of complications, and whatever else they thought would benefit the patient, but no personal contacts were made.

The experimental and control groups were similar to each other upon admission, but when the project ended, the group prayed for had statistically significantly better outcomes than the controls on cardiopulmonary arrest, congestive heart failure, pneumonia, diaretics, intubation/ventilation, and antibiotics. (Conditions outside the study like the prayers of relatives, friends, and clergy could not be controlled for either group.)

In a similar study of 990 patients admitted to the coronary care unit of St. Luke's Hospital in Kansas City, 524 were randomly assigned to a control group and 466 to a group prayed for separately as individuals by five of seventy-five volunteers. Neither the patients nor their physicians were aware of the study. The intercessors were from a variety of Christian traditions (35 percent nondenominational and 27 percent Episcopal, plus other Protestants and Roman Catholics). They were told only their patients' first names and asked to pray daily for twenty-eight days for their speedy recovery. Based upon thirty-five medical measurements, the patients prayed for did 11 percent better than those in the control group with statistical odds of about one in twenty-five that the difference could occur by chance alone (Harris et al., 1999).

Another study of 196 coronary artery bypass surgery graft patients at the University of Michigan Medical Center found that patients who prayed privately had better psychological outcomes one year after the surgery than those who did not. Other important coexisting factors were controlled, and the possibility that the effect of prayer stemmed merely from better affective conditions at the outset was ruled out. The authors concluded that bringing a spiritual dimension into health care for elderly adults "will help accomplish better functioning of . . . patients, and it may also contribute to substantial reduction in health care costs . . ." (Ai et al., 1998, p. 599).

The Judeo-Christian Scriptures include many passages about health, illness, and relationships between the body, mind, and spirit. These emphasize concepts of holiness, wholeness, and shalom that are closely related to those of sin and salvation. All center around the concept of the person as a unity or soul, not a collection of separable parts. Spiritual health and theology are closely related to mental health and psychology (see Malony, 1983; Anderson, 1998).

Spirituality and Mental Health

The relationships between spirituality and mental health are very complex. There are many measures of mental functioning and of spirituality, and both are inconsistently defined. When persons of intrinsic and extrinsic religiousness are lumped together in studies of religion in general, their opposite relationships with mental health cancel each other out. *Intrinsically religious* people internalize their faith and live it out regardless of consequences. They have higher self-esteem, better personality functioning, less paranoia, lower rates of depression, and less anxiety than the *extrinsically religious,* those who use religion only to obtain status, security, self-justification, health, or sociability. Taking all of the evidence into account, the best conclusion is that a healthy religious involvement is better for well-being than none (Richards and Bergin, 1997, pp. 78-86; Koenig, 1997, pp. 101-102; Koenig, 1995b, pp. 33-89). Evidence from several hundred studies confirms the conclusion that religious affiliation neither damages mental health nor fully predicts better mental health, but also that the correlations between religion and good mental health are strongest when the latter is carefully defined.

Findings are mixed about whether religion increases or decreases anxiety. About half of the studies objectively examining the question found an inverse relationship (as religiousness increases, anxiety decreases), but others discovered no relationship, and a few, nearly all of young adults, found a positive one (Koenig, 1994, pp. 250-255).

The Durham Veterans Administration Mental Health Survey discovered that religious coping is inversely related to depressive symptoms and major depressive disorders among hospitalized male patients. It was the only significant predictor of diminished depressive symptoms over time. A wide variety of other studies have similar findings (summarized in Koenig, 1994, pp. 144-246).

Elderly people are the most susceptible to loss of control over future events through bereavement, loss of friends and siblings, chronic illness, and their own death, all of which are strongly associated with depression. Yet the Yale Health and Aging Project discovered that religious involvement is directly related to reduced depression and modifies other important factors in depression (Idler, 1994, pp. 159-181). "Both cross-sectional and longitudinal studies now show that religious elders are less likely to become depressed when confronted with negative life events such as physical illness" (Koenig, 1995a, p. 24).

The Duke Epidemiologic Catchment Area study of 1,299 randomly selected community dwelling adults aged sixty and over found no evidence to support the theory that religion causes increased anxiety among devout persons, nor that it protected them from it or relieved it. However, the therapeutic effects of religion were masked by a turning to religion for comfort when other resources were lacking and by an attraction to religion among persons who were more prone to anxiety by temperament or intrapsychic conflicts (Koenig, 1994, pp. 255-275).

Qualifications of Health-Related Findings

The broadest systematic review to date covers over 325 studies on religion and physical health and nearly 800 on mental health. It found a preponderant relationship between greater religious involvement (variously measured) and better mental health, physical health, or lower use of health services (Koenig, McCullough, and Larson, 2000). To be sure, many of the research findings are correlational and must be taken with considerable reservation because

1. it is impossible and unethical to manipulate the spirituality of persons experimentally;
2. additional intervening variables that may influence spirituality and health are not controlled;
3. the necessary but difficult and expensive longitudinal studies are rare;
4. both spirituality and health are multidimensional; and
5. the measures are not highly refined.

However, the same reservations apply to research data on many other topics that are accepted in the social and behavioral sciences as "established truth."

Since about one-third of the U.S. population considers religion to be the most important factor in their lives and another one-third considers it to be an important influence, the impact of religion and spirituality on mental health ought not be ignored by researchers and practitioners (Richards and Bergin, 1997, pp. 84-85). We still need to differentiate among the various types of religion and discover the consequences of various faiths and their diverse theodicies to explain problems like illness, war, death, and other difficulties encountered in life (see Richards and Bergin, 1997, pp. 49-74; Clements, 1989). Research also is needed to distinguish the effects of pathological forms of religion and spirituality from those that are conventional (see Enroth, 1992; Koenig, 1997, pp. 104-111; Oates, 1955).

Significant ethical and theological issues are related to implementing research findings. What is the proper scope of professional services? Should physicians, social workers, and even clergy recommend that people change their religious and spiritual behavior? If research shows that people of one denomination are more healthful than those of others, should those who want better health change their affiliation? Does research linking religious/spiritual behavior with health impose the blame of moral failure upon many with poor health? (See Sloan, Bagiella, and Powell, 1999.) Would a mere change of outward affiliation and religious behavior without the conversion of an inner-faith conviction and spiritual commitment merely increase extrinsic religiousness and hypocrisy without bringing any health improvement?

As we examine the evidence on health and spirituality, the counsel of Linda George (Kauffman, 1998) about the need for caution also should be underscored: "The importance of religion for society and individuals is not going to rise or fall on what it does for health. We need to avoid the mentality that it just exists as a tool in the medicine chest to make people healthier" (p. 16).

Spirituality and Well-Being

Research on personal adjustment in old age began in the late 1940s. Several studies have shown relationships between life satisfaction, morale, successful aging, or related conceptualizations of total wellness and various aspects of religion and spirituality. With the rare exceptions of small, highly specialized groups and use of dubious religious measures, these have shown positive relationships—higher religious commitment and involvement are associated with higher life satisfaction or subjective well-being (Moberg, 1995).

Several studies show that elderly people draw upon religion when they are coping with illness, bereavement, anticipated death, and other adversities. More than younger people, they use spiritually based means of coping, seek support from clergy or church members, and use prayer, Bible reading, and other religious means to set their minds at ease with their problems. They are less likely to express discontent with God or their church. Their faith seems to operate as a stress buffer, distress deterrent, or stress suppressor. Although research on the subject is in its infancy, their faith seems to help them maintain and integrate the self, achieve mastery of a changing environment, come to grips with their finitude and death, achieve intimacy through the religious community, and reach closeness with God (Pargament, Van Haitsma, and Ensing, 1995; see Koenig, 1994). Black (1999) found that faith in God was a means of coping with hardship and enhancing self-esteem among elderly African-American women living in poverty. Their conversational petitionary prayers demonstrate a familiarity with God that releases them from despair in the belief that their hardship is part of a divine plan and that they will be rewarded in this life and the next.

Religious conversion, defined by Koenig (1994) as "a profound reorientation of goals and motivations in life so that God (or Jesus for the Christian) becomes the object of ultimate concern" (p. 436), often occurs in mid and late life. Koenig claims that 40 percent of elderly men experience such changes in religious faith after the age of fifty. Except for persons who already had serious psychiatric illness prior to conversion, no research "documents an induction of mental illness by religious conversion in previously stable individuals" (p. 434). On the contrary, conversion increases well-being, resolves depression, frees from alcohol abuse, decreases anxiety, decreases selfishness, expands the desire to help others, and implants a new sense of purpose and hope (pp. 419-438).

Most studies show that higher religiousness and spirituality are associated with lower levels of death anxiety, less alcoholism, fewer suicides, better marriages, greater adaptation to Alzheimer's disease caregiving, reduced loneliness, hopefulness among disabled elders, and general mental health (Koenig, 1995b, pp. 73-89). This, of course, is no excuse for physical barriers to participation in religious congregations, nor for youth-valuing stereotypes and negative myths about aging that demean elder members. It does not validate deficiencies of clergy for their ministries with aging people nor defend their ignoring other problems many older people encounter in their religious organizations (Moberg, 1997; see Gray and Moberg, 1977, pp. 121-140).

CONCLUSION

This chapter summarized the overwhelming evidence from research that high levels of religiousness and spirituality are correlated positively with life satisfaction, health, healing, and well-being. Findings scattered throughout other chapters of this book supply additional evidence of similar relationships. The consistency of the findings is similar to a form of construct validity in which the predominant results of each measurement are consistent with the results of others. However, most of the research is based upon samples of American people whose heritage, if not also their current orientations, is mainly in Christianity, and the measures of spirituality are directly or indirectly derived from Christian values. Although most elderly Americans today share that heritage, the scene is changing, so a much broader range of research is needed (see Chapters 15 and 16).

REFERENCES

Ai, Amy L., Ruth E. Dunkle, Christopher Peterson, and Steven F. Bolling (1998). The role of private prayer in psychological recovery among midlife and aged patients following cardiac surgery. *The Gerontologist* 38(5):591-601.

Anderson, Ray S. (1998). On being human: The spiritual saga of a creaturely soul. In Brown, Warren S., Nancey Murphy, and H. Newton Malony (Eds.), *Whatever happened to the soul?: Scientific and theological portraits of human nature* (pp. 175-194). Minneapolis, MN: Fortress Press.

Black, Helen K. (1999). Poverty and prayer: Spiritual narratives of elderly African-American women. *Review of Religious Research* 40(4):359-374.

Byrd, Randall C. (1988). Positive therapeutic effects of intercessory prayer in a coronary care unit population. *Southern Medical Journal* 81(7):826-829.

Carson, Verna Benner (1989). *Spiritual dimensions of nursing practice.* Philadelphia: W. B. Saunders Co.

Clements, William M. (Ed.) (1989). *Religion, aging and health: A global perspective* (compiled by the World Health Organization). Binghamton, NY: The Haworth Press.

Ellor, James W. (1997). America now and into the 21st century: Generations aging together with independence. *Aging and Religion* 2(1):1-11.

Enroth, Ronald M. (1992). *Churches that abuse.* Grand Rapids, MI: Zondervan Publishing House.

Gray, Robert M. and David O. Moberg (1977). *The church and the older person* (revised edition). Grand Rapids, MI: Eerdmans.

Harris, William S., Manohar Gowda, Jerry W. Kolb, Christopher P. Strychacz, James L. Vacek, Philip G. Jones, Alan Forker, James H. O'Keefe, and Ben D. McCallister (1999). A randomized, controlled trial of the effects of remote, intercessory prayer on outcomes in patients admitted to the coronary care unit. *Archives of Internal Medicine* 159(19):2273-2278.

Hill, Peter C. and Ralph W. Hood Jr. (Eds.) (1999). *Measures of religiosity.* Birmingham, AL: Religious Education Press.

Hummer, Robert A., Richard G. Rogers, Charles B. Nam, and Christopher G. Ellison (1999). Religious involvement and U.S. adult mortality. *Demography* 36(2):273-285.

Idler, Ellen L. (1994). *Cohesiveness and coherence: Religion and the health of the elderly.* New York: Garland Publishing, Inc.

Kauffman, Dan (1998). Does religious participation and commitment relate to recovery from illness?: An interview with Linda K. George. *Science & Spirit* 9(5, December):16.

Koenig, Harold G. (1994). *Aging and God: Spiritual pathways to mental health in midlife and later years.* Binghamton, NY: The Haworth Pastoral Press.

Koenig, Harold G. (1995a). Religion and health in later life. In Kimble, Melvin A., Susan H. McFadden, James W. Ellor, and James J. Seeber (Eds.), *Aging, spirituality, and religion* (pp. 9-29). Minneapolis, MN: Fortress Press.

Koenig, Harold G. (1995b). *Research on religion and aging: An annotated bibliography.* Westport, CT: Greenwood Press.

Koenig, Harold G. (1997). *Is religion good for your health? The effects of religion on physical and mental health.* Binghamton, NY: The Haworth Press.

Koenig, Harold G. and David B. Larson (1998). Use of hospital services, religious attendance, and religious affiliation. *Southern Medical Journal* 91(10):925-932.

Koenig, Harold G., Michael E. McCullough, and David B. Larson (Eds.) (2000). *Handbook of religion and health: A century of research reviewed.* New York: Oxford University Press.

Koenig, Harold G., Mona Smiley, and Jo Ann Ploch Gonzales (1988). *Religion, health, and aging: A review and theoretical integration.* Westport, CT: Greenwood Press.

Levin, Jeffrey S. (1994). Introduction. In Levin, Jeffrey S. (Ed.), *Religion in aging and health: Theoretical foundations and methodological frontiers* (pp. xv-xxiv). Thousand Oaks, CA: Sage Publications.

Levin, Jeffrey S. (1995). "Epidemiology of religion." Paper presented at the April conference of the National Institute for Healthcare Research, Leesburg, VA.

Malony, H. Newton (Ed.) (1983). *Wholeness and holiness: Readings in the psychology/theology of mental health.* Grand Rapids, MI: Baker Book House.

Mindel, C. H. and Vaughan, C. E. (1978). A multidimensional approach to religiosity and disengagement. *Journal of Gerontology* 33(1):103-108.

Moberg, David O. (1979). The development of social indicators for quality of life research. *Sociological Analysis* 40(1):11-26.

Moberg, David O. (1995). Applications of research methods. In Kimble, Melvin A., Susan H. McFadden, James W. Ellor, and James J. Seeber (Eds.), *Aging, spirituality, and religion* (pp. 541-557). Minneapolis, MN: Fortress Press.

Moberg, David O. (1997). Religion and aging. In Ferraro, Kenneth F. (Ed.), *Gerontology: Perspectives and issues,* Second edition (pp. 193-220). New York: Springer Publishing Co.

Moberg, David O. (1999). The Great Commission and research. *Perspectives on Science and Christian Faith* 51(1):8-16.

Moody, Harry R. (1994). Foreword: The Owl of Minerva. In Thomas, L. Eugene and Susan A. Eisenhandler (Eds.), *Aging and the human dimension* (pp. ix-xv). Westport, CT: Auburn House.

Oates, Wayne (1955). *Religious factors in mental illness.* New York: Association Press.

Pargament, Kenneth I., Kimberly S. Van Haitsma, and David S. Ensing (1995). Religion and coping. In Kimble, Melvin A., Susan H. McFadden, James W. Ellor, and James J. Seeber (Eds.), *Aging, spirituality, and religion* (pp. 47-67). Minneapolis, MN: Fortress Press.

Richards, P. Scott and Allen E. Bergin (1997). *A spiritual strategy for counseling and psychotherapy.* Washington, DC: American Psychological Association.

Shelly, Judith Allen and Sharon Fish (1988). *Spiritual care: The nurse's role,* Third edition. Downers Grove, IL: InterVarsity Press.

Sloan, R. P., E. Bagiella, and T. Powell (1999). Religion, spirituality, and medicine. *Lancet* 353(9153):664-667.

Chapter 5

Attitudes Toward Death and Dying Among Persons in the Fourth Quarter of Life

Joanne Armatowski, SSND

As human beings, we have always been concerned with death. We have developed rituals, designed institutions, formulated concepts, and constructed language to help us cope with our mortality and ultimate death. This awareness is a part of the aging process (Kalish, 1985, p. 27). For most adults in the fourth quarter of life (those over age seventy-five), death awareness embodies the meaning of aging in its spiritual dimension. Death is as much a part of human existence and of human growth and development as being born.

The purpose of this chapter, therefore, is to identify and examine the research on attitudes toward death and dying among persons in the fourth quarter of life. As part of the process, I interviewed six elderly religious sisters and will present their views on spirituality and how it relates to their own preparation for dying.

ATTITUDES TOWARD DEATH THROUGHOUT HISTORY

From the early Middle Ages until the mid-nineteenth century, the attitude toward death in Western civilization was almost static; changes occurred slowly and often went unnoticed. Today changes are more rapid and perceptible. The last two-thirds of the twentieth century witnessed a revolution in traditional ideas and feelings about death. In the past, death was omnipresent and familiar, a common occurrence in the family situation (Aries, 1974, p. 57). At the same time, death was considered mysterious and was celebrated with ceremony.

This evolution accelerated between 1930 and 1950. Up to that time, people died at home, and the wakes and cultural and family traditions were carried out in the home. Changes occurred mainly when most people no longer died at home with family and friends nearby, but in a hospital and often alone. Death was no longer part of peoples' daily consciousness. During this period, consequently, many of the rites and rituals of death and dying were discontinued (Aries, 1974, p. 87).

The continuing advances of medical technology have altered attitudes toward dying. They compel a reexamination of death from the standpoint of honored traditions and community supports. Because death is for everyone and for all seasons of life, people on the far end of the chronological continuum or old age, want to share their feelings and thoughts about dying and death. They are frequently prohibited from doing so because of our general reluctance to examine death (Feifel, 1977, p. 42). A result of this reluctance is that far too many elderly persons exhibit repressive and inappropriate behaviors in dealing with their fears and hopes about death.

DEFINITIONS OF DYING AND DEATH

The literature defines dying and death from a number of perspectives, many of which depend on people's belief systems. Three of the most common definitions of dying are as follows:

- Dying is a journey a person must take in the last phase of life. It is the process leading to the end and, for older persons, it can sometimes be a long journey of progressive suffering on many levels. They often fear weakness, pain, physical dependence, and mental deterioration more than the cessation of life (Fischer, 1998, p. 163).
- The dying stage in our life can be experienced as the most profound growth event of our total life's experience (Kübler-Ross, 1975, p. 149).

- Dying is an interactive process. Dying begins when the facts are recognized. Dying begins when the facts are communicated. Dying begins when the patient realizes or accepts the facts (Kastenbaum, 1986, pp. 90-91).

The corresponding definitions of death follow:

- Death is the final moment of life, the end of life as we know it (Fischer, 1998, p. 163).
- Death is the final stage of growth in this life. There is no total death. Only the body dies. The self or spirit, or whatever you may wish to label it, is eternal. You may interpret this in any way that makes you comfortable (Kübler-Ross, 1975, p. 166).
- Death is the nonreversible cessation of the life process (Kastenbaum, 1986, p. 17).

ATTITUDES TOWARD DYING AND DEATH

Behavioral scientists began scientific studies of death only about thirty years ago. Because death transcends old age, major research during this period focused on children, adolescents, adults, and the elderly. Most of the research on dying and death has fallen into two categories: studies probing emotions or attitudes surrounding death and investigations exploring the experience of dying itself.

The focus here is on the elderly who often have extensive experiences dealing with death. Most elderly persons recognize that their own death is close at this time in their lives. It is assumed by a number of behavioral scientists that older people must think about dying and death more than any other age group does (Belsky, 1990, p. 327).

Authors and a variety of studies revealed, especially in the last twenty years, that a number of attitudes toward dying and death could refer to most age groups but are most often depicted in the elderly. A discussion of these attitudes follows.

Attitude: Fear of Dying and Death

Most researchers consider "attitudes toward death" and "fear of death" as synonymous. Feifel and Branscomb (1973) found through the use of a death perspective scale that was later described by Spilka and colleagues (1977, p. 174) that older people were less fearful of death on the conscious than they are on the unconscious level. In the study by Templer, Ruff, and Franks (1971), however, there was no relationship between age and fear of death. Other studies have also produced conflicting findings about the relationship between age and fear of death.

Present research reveals that it is difficult to know how older people genuinely feel about death. While that fear may diminish in later life, it does not disappear. Approximately 50 to 75 percent of older adults experience fear or anxiety about death (Koenig, 1994, p. 44).

Denying any fear of death may be a sign of great inner turmoil. The elderly may have more fear of death than they will admit. Yet, when questioned, they admit that they fear the dying process more than death itself. Many are concerned with the suffering of intense pain and of having what they call "the humiliation" of depending on others. Other aspects of fear revolve around questions like "Who will care for me in my final days?" and "Will I suffer greatly, be in unbearable pain, and be a burden to those I love?"

Evidence of the relationship between religious conviction and fear of death are inconclusive even today, although a number of authors believe that there is a positive correlation between death attitudes and religious convictions as they are related to the fear of death. The concept of certainty or uncertainty about what happens after death seems to provide meaning to the elderly. This was assessed by behavioral scientists through a subscale of questions regarding "death as afterlife-of-reward" (Smith, Nehemkis, and Charter, 1983; Fischer, 1998, p. 196).

Attitude: Hope

All humans face growing old, but are unable to concretely imagine their own dying process. They are also unable to see themselves as truly old because for most people the change is frightening. As a result, the spirituality of aging will remain shallow unless they dwell in some depth on the special and threatening problems of old age (Bianchi, 1982, p. 131). The journey for each person is individual.

Therefore, no single type of religiousness will satisfy a person confronting old age. Some find help in liturgical practices, others in social gospel activities, some in mysticism, and others in a combination of these and other forms of spirituality. Every person discovers this path and often in this discovery recognizes the continuity of hope with the past (Kalish, 1985, p. 59).

Even though hope lies at the center of every human life, the elderly often experience hopelessness. This could evolve from an overextension of hope, an attitude that leaves no room for any expressions of discouragement and imposes an impossible ideal on elderly persons. People need to realize that expressions of anger can coexist with love, as can despair with hope. If this is not recognized, it burdens people with a sense that they ought to have only beautiful feelings, which in turn leaves no room for some of the rage that is buried within them. A valid and honest hope takes into account the harsh realities that people experience both personally and in the world (Fischer, 1998, p. 132).

Hope enables all, including the elderly, to see things from a different perspective. It challenges persons to weave the pieces of life into new patterns or to shine a new light on something old. Christians often find comforting hope-filled words in the Scriptures.

Attitude: Loss

Loss is a constant theme in writings and reflections on dying and death: "What do I lose when I am dying?" "What will I have lost when I am dead?" Many losses accompany the dying process and death itself. Some of the losses discussed in research are the loss of experiencing, the loss of people, the loss of control and competence, the loss of capacity to complete projects and plans, the loss of body capabilities, and the loss of dreams for the future.

These losses may be mainly external, but they are often internalized and diminish the self-image. One grieves not only for the losses, but also for the ultimate loss of self. For example, the loss of friends and family members and the loss of work through retirement frequently cause people to lose their sense of worth or usefulness. They are experiencing a time in life when they are less able to change because of social and personal diminishments. Yet, at this time, they are often required to make severe changes in their jobs, housing and status (Bianchi, 1982, p. 156).

Dealing with these losses is one of the greatest spiritual challenges of aging. Losses occur throughout life, but they often come at a faster pace during the last years. Some of the losses that presently accompany aging may be lessened or even eliminated in the future because of advances in medical science. How loss is handled is one of the most critical factors in the happiness or unhappiness of the elderly person.

The biblical story of the account of Israel's experience of exile clearly identifies three movements that are particularly important for understanding and living through losses with faith. They are (1) a new song in a foreign land, (2) every morning God's mercies are new, and (3) God will never forget you (Fischer, 1998, pp. 146-158). As one deals with the losses that accompany aging, this story can enlighten and strengthen a person.

Attitude: Dignity/Integrity

In order to preserve their dignity, integrity, and self-worth, the elderly need to know that others support them. The supportive task of others is simply to see the beauty that lies within, accept the truth of who and what they in essence are, and capture the goodness. This acceptance often leads to humility, which is another form of being honest in accepting the truth (Johnson, 1992).

Helping others, whenever possible, will strengthen and complete, rather than weaken and fragment, the lives of those who care. Giving love enables individuals to recognize and be grateful for the love that God gives to them every day. This type of positive attitude has a direct impact on other persons and allows all to realize more clearly the central life-sustaining fact of existence—that all are children of God. This stewardship will allow humanity to achieve all that it is possible to achieve even in late life (Valentine, 1994, p. 74).

Attitude: Forgiveness

Forgiveness means ceasing to feel any claim to recompense. It requires an emphatic healing of memories (Bianchi, 1982, p. 66). A person forgives in order to bring peace into one's own life. Through this human process, persons are caught up in the forgiveness of God, which enables them to forgive.

For most people, the most motivational benefits that occur from forgiving are exemplified in practical ways. Forgiveness stimulates new spiritual and emotional growth in a person. By letting go of blame, one releases energy that is trapped in the unproductive service of holding a grudge and unleashes it for use in growth-filled ways.

Difficult as it is, forgiving others is still easier than forgiving oneself (Beha, 1997). All humans sin and continue to sin into old age. Yet, all are called to accept forgiveness and the opportunity to learn new and loving behaviors. The first step is to recognize personal behaviors, failure to love, and the need to change.

Another step to receiving forgiveness is to tell another human being. This is a way of admitting the need to learn how to love. It also enables one to admit the need for help from God and at times from other human beings.

In later life, this is of special concern. The hurts and failures of the past can suddenly flood one with so many unhealed and unresolved remembrances that one may feel overwhelmed by them. Guilt and bitterness could result from failure to forgive one's self and others (Thibault, 1993, p. 121). On the other hand, one needs to keep in mind that the outcome of repentance is forgiveness. One asks for forgiveness and the ability to let go of guilt.

Attitude: Loneliness

Loneliness is the painful experience that happens as a result of partial or total dissatisfaction with the human longings for contact, communication, and companionship. Loneliness is such a painful experience for some people that they would do practically anything to avoid it. It is the experience of not being meaningfully related to oneself, to significant others, to the earth, or ultimately to God.

The older person does not want to be a burden to others but, on the other hand, often carries a heavy burden. Before the person is able to work through the death of a loved one, another may die; and typically, there is not much opportunity for distraction through work or other activities. Some of the consequences of loneliness are loss of appetite, insomnia, depression, and other common components of the grief response. These can have serious consequences for a person who is already suffering from age-related health problems (Feifel, 1977, p. 41).

Another aspect of loneliness is isolation. It is important to avoid social isolation as much as possible. One needs to continue to evaluate one's degree of involvement with family and friends. If one is able to identify the factors that contribute to social isolation, one is able to develop strategies to reduce social isolation and reengage in social life (Doka, 1993, p. 103).

In reflecting on loneliness, it is important to note the difference between loneliness and aloneness. Creative solitude is a positive path that defines the experience of aloneness. Further, solitude, whether in aloneness or in company with others, is a feeling of letting one's self be, without forcing or controlling events (Bianchi, 1982, p. 49). Old age necessarily entails a unique aloneness that is proper to this time in life. The challenge is not to run away from loneliness and aloneness, for it can be "the key to spiritual life."

Attitude: Love

Growth in love is the perennial challenge in every age of the human person. Love not only opens individuals to the mystery of human life but also reveals God to them. Older people are frequently told that it does not matter if their productivity declines with age since lasting self-worth is grounded in God's love. While this is true, it is difficult to experience unless God's love is mediated through genuine human love from others. The Gospel calls all to deepen and expand the quality of their love during the later years.

Social scientists today are exploring more fully several aspects of love in later life, especially in three major areas: love and sex after sixty, the importance of friendship in the later years, and the call to compassion and universal love. Love in these later years usually is not displayed on a dramatic scale (Fischer, 1998, p. 89).

The attitudes presented here are some of the most prominent ones found in the research literature. Others, such as personal identity, sense of worth, regret, grief, and gratitude, are not mentioned often in current research literature. All are important and need to be researched further in light of the spiritual needs of persons in the fourth quarter of life.

TYPES OF SPIRITUALITY DEFINITIONS

In reflecting on the attitudes of persons, especially those in the fourth quarter of life, it is evident that all these people have spiritual needs. From the above summary, I gleaned three foundational spiritual needs: meaning and purpose of life, unconditional love, and the experience of forgiveness. These are essential for a person's spiritual well-being.

Further research on dying and death emphasizes a realization of the importance of spirituality and spiritual well-being. The wording of the definitions varies, but the essence of their meanings remains constant. The following definitions provide a basis for understanding the comments that were shared by the six religious women whom I interviewed.

Spirituality—All of Life

Spirituality means not just one compartment of life, but the deepest dimension of all of life. The spiritual is the ultimate ground of all our questions, hopes, fears, and loves. It includes our efforts to deal creatively with retirement and to find purpose in our lives after our family has been raised. It concerns our struggles with the loss of a spouse or the move from a home of many years, our questions of self-worth and the fear of reaching out to make new friendships, and our discovery of new talents, deeper peace, wider boundaries of love. All these are spiritual concerns. Christian spirituality involves the entire human person in all of his or her relationships (Fischer, 1998, p. 13).

Spirituality—Relationship

Spirituality is the consciousness and awareness of a relationship with the Lord, together with a modification of one's attitudes and behavior in light of that relationship (Fahey, 1991).

Spirituality—Meaning in Life

Spirituality is not only the conscious religious disciplines and practices through which human beings relate to God, but more inclusively, the whole style and meaning of our relationship to that which we perceive as of ultimate worth and power (Nelson, 1983, p. 5).

Work on spiritual well-being complements the above definitions and indicates other important aspects of spirituality during the fourth quarter of life. The most widely used definition for over twenty-five years is the ecumenical definition created by the National Interfaith Coalition on Aging in 1975. It states:

> Spiritual well-being is the affirmation of life in a relationship with God, self, community, and environment that nurtures and celebrates wholeness. (Seeber, 1990, p. 6)

Another definition that encompasses the breadth of spiritual well-being states:

> Spiritual well-being embraces and encompasses all of our relationships that have meaning in our lives from our past, present, and future. (Murphy, 1991, p. 18)

INTERVIEWS ON DEATH, DYING, AND SPIRITUALITY

After reading and studying the research on death, dying, and spirituality, I decided to interview six religious sisters from the School Sisters of Notre Dame. Each interview lasted approximately one hour. The sisters were given four questions one week before the interview. The questions were sent prior to their appointment time so they could reflect and focus on the three issues of death, dying, and spirituality.

The women interviewed ranged in age from seventy-five to ninety: two were in their seventies, three in their eighties, and one had just turned ninety. All are Catholic sisters who have been in religious life for at least fifty years, and most between sixty and seventy years. All possess master's degrees or beyond. They reside in Elm Grove, Wisconsin, in an assisted living facility with 150 residents (all sisters) who range in age from fifty to ninety-nine years.

For purposes of this chapter, I will share only the key concepts that each sister incorporated into her answers to the four questions. (The questions in the letter sent to them led to a number of other personal stories that are only partially reflected in this chapter.) The following are summaries of their responses.

Do you feel that you have become more religious as you have grown older?

All six of the sisters connected "religious" with obligations, rules, laws, a framework, and confinement. One went a step further and defined "religious" as "placing undue importance on the nonessentials" (this was the ninety-year-old who has written books and given presentations on the elderly and aging).

How would you describe your own spirituality and your own spiritual life?

The sisters all responded with "simple" and in various terms spoke of their relationship with God and others. Externals did not seem important to them at this time in their lives. Living in the "now," the present moment, and recognizing that spirituality continues to deepen as one ages is key for each of them. Their prayer was one of "Yes, Lord; Take, Lord, receive"; and "Fiat," which to them means to say "yes" to God's will.

What is your perception of death? Your attitudes toward death?

Because of their beliefs, the sisters replied with similar answers. Two of the six sisters' perceived death as inevitable and an ending, while the others perceived it as a new beginning, a movement in life, a process, and a shock, a change as much as birth. Even though there seemed to be a fear of "how death would come," the sisters' attitudes were positive. Their responses consisted of living today in readiness for God, hope for the afterlife, awareness of the death of family and friends, and recognition that letting go was most difficult.

Are you afraid to die? Why or why not?

This last question seemed to be the source of the most reflection for the sisters. All six did claim that they did not fear death itself. Two specifically indicated that they would welcome death. All six indicated that they are ready to die and agree that this is what they lived for all their lives as women of faith. It is the process of dying that some feared more than others. Each one has her struggles and questions with the dying process. As one admitted: "Some days I am at peace and welcome death and other days I struggle with the diminishment." Because they are women of faith, prayer and reflection often comfort them in times of struggle.

SUMMARY

Research since the 1960s is inconclusive regarding attitudes toward dying and death during the fourth quarter of life. From all that I have read, the one aspect that stands out clearly is fear of the dying process. It seems that most of the elderly in this period of their lives are not afraid of death itself but of all that could precede death.

The interviews with Catholic sisters reveal that spirituality for them is simple and focuses on self, others, and the world. The process of dying and death is unique to each individual, but the attitudes discussed above are basic to most Christians, whether young or elderly. The elderly, in most cases, think about dying and death more often and come face to face with death more frequently because of the deaths of family and friends.

In moving through both the positive and negative attitudes of dying and death, persons (not all) eventually come to peace after a struggle of letting go. As a society, we, especially Americans, shy away from death and endings. In recent years research has led people toward greater awareness and more study of the dying process and death. Even though the elderly in the fourth quarter of life fear the dying process, I believe that they view death as a necessary step to something better.

CONCLUSION

Researchers will continue to observe the lives of the elderly who have a legacy to share by their living and dying. Many persons have gifted us with that legacy. One who has done just that in a thought-provoking manner for me is the late Cardinal Joseph Bernadin (McClury, 1999) as he wrote on November 14, 1994, three weeks before his death from terminal cancer:

> I am at peace and I can only account for that by looking upon it as a gift from God. . . . First of all, you really have to trust the Lord. . . . The second thing is that if you believe the Lord and trust the Lord, you should be able to see death as a friend, and not as an enemy. If the first is right and the second is right, the third follows: you have to let go. That letting go is not the easiest thing in the world. (p. 10)

REFERENCES

Aries, P. (1974). *Western attitudes toward death.* Baltimore: The Johns Hopkins University Press.

Beha, Marie (1997). Seventy and counting. *Review for Religious* 56(3):302-310.

Belsky, Janet K. (1990). *The psychology of aging* (Second edition). Pacific Grove, CA: Brooks/Cole Publishing Company.

Bianchi, Eugene C. (1982). *Aging as a spiritual journey.* New York: Crossroad Publishing Company.

Doka, K. (1993). *Living with life-threatening illness.* New York: Lexington Books.

Fahey, Charles (1991). Why we need a spirituality of aging. *St. Anthony Messenger* 6(1):16-21.

Feifel, H. (1977). *New meanings of death.* New York: McGraw-Hill Book Company.

Feifel, H. and A. Branscomb (1973). Who's afraid of death? *Journal of Abnormal Psychology* 81(2):282-288.

Fischer, Kathleen (1998). *Winter grace.* Nashville: Upper Room Books.

Johnson, R. (1992). Forgiveness: Our bridge to peace. *Liguorian* 80(6)(June):44-45.

Kalish, R. (1985). *Death, grief, and caring relationships* (Second edition). Monterey, CA: Brooks/Cole Publishing Company.

Kastenbaum, Robert J. (1986). *Death, society, and human experience* (Third edition). Columbus, OH: Charles E. Merrill Publishing Company.

Koenig, Harold (1994). *Aging and God.* Binghamton, New York: The Haworth Press.

Kübler-Ross, Elisabeth (1975). *Death: The final stage of growth.* New York: Simon & Schuster, Inc.

McClury, Robert (1999). Faithful departures: How Catholics face the end of life. *U.S. Catholic* 1(1):10-16.

Murphy, Pat (1991). Why we need a spirituality of aging. *St. Anthony Messenger* 6(1):16-21.

Nelson, J. (1983). *Between two gardens: Reflections on sexuality and religious experience.* New York: Pilgrim Press.

Seeber, James J. (Ed.). (1990). *Spiritual maturity in the later years.* Binghamton, New York: The Haworth Press.

Smith, D., A. Nehemkis, and R. Charter (1983). Fear of death, death attitudes, and religious conviction in the terminally ill. *International Journal of Psychiatry in Medicine* 13(3):221-231.

Spilka, B., L. Stout, B. Milton, and D. Sizemore (1977). Death and personal faith: A psychometric investigation. *Journal for the Scientific Study of Religion* 16(1):169-178.

Templer, D., C. Ruff, and C. Franks (1971). Death anxiety: Age, sex and parental resemblance in diverse populations. *Developmental Psychology* 4(1):108-112.

Thibault, Jane M. (1993). *A deepening love affair: The gift of God in later life.* Nashville: Upper Room Books.

Valentine, Mary Hester (1994). *Aging in the Lord.* New York: Paulist Press.

Chapter 6

Do Spirituality and Religiosity Increase with Age?

Pamela Lynn Schultz-Hipp

As people progress through their life stages, religion often becomes a strongly integrated part of their lives. Does this change include increased spirituality? And is it a result of the aging process or simply an expression of membership in an age cohort that is more religious than the younger age groups?

Psychologist Starbuck (1911) concluded that people do tend to become more spiritual as they age and that their "faith and belief in God grow in importance as the years advance" (as quoted by Baker and Nussbaum, 1997, p. 34). However, continuity theory (see Chapter 3, this volume) and researchers such as Hall (1922), Cavan and colleagues (1949), Orbach (1961), and Palmore (1980) have concluded that people do not grow more religious as they age. The longitudinal studies by Blazer and Palmore (1976) also suggest that religious satisfaction and attitudes tend not to change after age seventeen.

On the other hand, Stokes (1990) has shown that spirituality is not static. "Faith development does not occur at a consistent rate or in a uniform way throughout adulthood, but rather in varying patterns of activity and quiescence directly related to specific chronological periods of the adult life cycle" (p. 176). A change in spirituality or religiousness could be the result of an individual's life experiences, not only of various cohort effects.

CONCEPTS OF SPIRITUALITY

Spirituality is the human awareness of a relationship or connection that goes beyond sensory perceptions. This relationship, as perceived by each person, is an expanded or heightened knowledge beyond or outside of his or her personal being. This knowledge is not controlled by the subject's efforts; instead it is given substance by drawing on the person's life experiences for its shape and substance.

Spirituality was eloquently defined by Holmes (1982) as "a human capacity for relationship with that which transcends sense phenomena" (p. 12). A person perceives it as a heightened or expanded consciousness that is independent of one's efforts and that deepens one's awareness of self, others, and world. A deepened awareness of the Holy exhibits itself in creative action in the world.

Holmes' (1982) phenomenological description of spirituality is generic, not restricted to any specific religion. The historic setting of a person in a geographic location and a network of employment, political commitments, family, and other social relationships provides the matrix within which spirituality is formed and developed. But from a Christian perspective, it must include relationships with fellow believers in a community that shapes personal spirituality through the Word, sacraments, traditions, rituals, and symbols that nurture one's relation with the Transcendent (God).

When we think of the Word and Sacrament, rituals, traditions, and symbols, we think of religion. "An ultimate function of religion is to provide meaning for life" (Rogers, 1976, p. 415). One's destiny is really defined as life because destiny is popularly defined as "that which was meant to be." Something within you knows who you are and what you are supposed to be. That "something" refers to a destiny that is written into the structure of one's being (Johnson, 1989). When people reach the later stages of life (for our purposes defined as sixty-five and older), they question whether or not they have fulfilled their life purpose. The answer to this question, more often than not, directs the aged person back to his or her own religious beliefs. "As long as a man lives, he must believe in something for the sake of which he lives; without belief in something that makes life worth living man cannot exist" (Niebuhr, 1967, p. 56).

The ability to give one's loyalty and to place one's trust in God or something transcendent is faith. A person must cling to the centers of value and faith that fill the mold of spirituality and cultivate the God/self relationship. This relationship is nurtured through personal and community worship and integrated into meditations on scripture or other spiritual writings, sacraments, and retreats. When these rituals are executed with a whole heart, the transcendence of the God/self relationship is strengthened and spirituality soars.

THE IMPORTANCE
OF RELIGION TO OLDER ADULTS

Differences in religion do exist between age groups (Moberg, 1997). Findings from various Gallup Polls in 1993 show that among adults under age thirty only 32 percent attended church or synagogue in a typical week compared with 52 percent of those age sixty-five and older, far more of whom feel religion is very important in their own lives compared to adults younger than sixty-five.

> The general pattern of highest religiosity among the elderly on almost all measures has remained the same year after year when similar questions are asked. They are confirmed by parallel findings from other national polls. For example, the 1993 and 1994 surveys of the Barna Research Group (Barna, 1994) showed that respondents aged sixty-seven-plus were more likely than young and middle-aged Americans to believe that . . . religion is very important in their lives. (Moberg, 1997, p. 195)

Religion and spirituality are so important in the later years that aging has been referred to as "a spiritual journey" (Bianchi, 1984) and "a spiritualizing process" (Jones, 1984; see Moberg, 1990). Professionals who work with aging families can help them explore their spiritual tasks of facing mortality, defining the shape and limits of love and fidelity, struggling with the meaning of evil and suffering, seeking forgiveness and reconciliation, and giving plus receiving a spiritual legacy (Fischer, 1992).

AGE DIFFERENCES AMONG WOMEN AT A LUTHERAN RETREAT

To discover whether women past age sixty-five differ from those who are younger, a short, anonymous questionnaire was distributed to 784 women from all parts of Wisconsin who attended a Christian women's retreat on March 12 to 15, 1999, that was organized by a Wisconsin Evangelical Lutheran Synod congregation. Although the research was not sponsored by the retreat staff, 650 questionnaires (83 percent) were returned. Only four were from persons under age twenty, ninety-one (13 percent) were ages twenty to thirty-four, 306 (47 percent) ages thirty-five to forty-nine, 181 (27 percent) ages fifty to sixty-four, and seventy-one (10 percent) ages sixty-five or older. Only 6 percent were single, 5 percent were divorced or separated, 7 percent widowed, and the remaining 81 percent were married.

Although the retreat was open to women of any religion, fewer than 3 percent of the respondents were non-Lutherans, and nearly all the Lutherans were from the Wisconsin Synod (see Table 6.1). In answer to the question, "What denomination would you say your core beliefs are most closely associated with?", very few mentioned one different from their own.

TABLE 6.1. Religious Core Beliefs versus Religious Denomination

CORE BELIEFS	RELIGION	RELIGIOUS DENOMINATION
1.23%	Catholic	1.07%
.61%	Evangelical Lutheran	.31%
4.30%	Missouri Synod Lutheran	2.29%
91.09%	Wisconsin Evangelical Lutheran	94.50%
.77%	Baptist	.15%
.31%	Methodist	.46%
.46%	Pentecostal	.15%
.15%	Presbyterian	.15%
1.08%	Other	.92%

In response to the question, "How often do you attend worship services?", there is a direct relationship with age (see Table 6.2). Although nearly all of the women attended once or more per week, those past age sixty-five (94 percent weekly) and those aged fifty to sixty-four (95 percent) attended slightly more frequently than those aged thirty-five to forty (91 percent) and younger than thirty-five (85 percent).

The frequency of private prayer shows a similar pattern (see Table 6.3). Of the women past sixty-five, 94 percent prayed daily or more often, compared to 87 percent of those aged fifty to sixty-four, 85 percent of those aged thirty-five to forty-nine, and 75 percent of the younger women. (Whether the prayers were predominately praise and thanksgiving, petition for their own needs, intercession for others, imprecations, or some other types or combinations of types was not asked.)

TABLE 6.2. How Often Do You Attend Worship Services?

	Under 35 Years	35-49 Years	50-64 Years	65+ Years
More Than 1 Time Per Week	19.79%	23.47%	34.40%	35.21%
About 1 Time Per Week	65.98%	67.20%	61.11%	59.15%
2 or 3 Times Per Month	11.34%	7.07%	2.78%	4.23%
About 1 Time Per Month	3.09%	.96%	.56%	0
A Few Times Per Year	0	.96%	1.11%	1.41%
Never	0	.32%	0	0
TOTAL	100%	100%	100%	100%

TABLE 6.3. How Often Do You Pray Privately?

	Under 35 Years	35-49 Years	50-64 Years	65+ Years
Several Times Each Day	37.50%	52.41%	62.43%	59.15%
Daily	37.50%	32.80%	24.86%	35.21%
Several Times Each Week	18.75%	9.97%	9.39%	1.41%
Occasionally	6.25%	4.82%	2.76%	1.41%
Only in Crisis/Emergency	0	0	0	2.82%
Never	0	0	.56%	0
TOTAL	100%	100%	100%	100%

Table 6.4 summarizes their answers to the question, "How important are your religious beliefs?". Although nearly all of these retreat respondents considered their religion extremely or very important to themselves, the oldest women had the highest proportion (86 percent) saying it was extremely important.

Because those of all ages who attended this retreat were so highly religious, the age differences in the expressions of religion and spirituality that were measured are minimal. However, they are consistently in the direction of highest levels among the oldest age group, as has been observed with few exceptions in study after study elsewhere. Such cross-sectional findings that simply compare people of different ages do not demonstrate changes over time, although the consistency of the relationship over several decades is strong circumstantial evidence of a possible trend, especially if we agree that American society itself is characterized by increasing levels of secularization.

TABLE 6.4. How Important Are Your Religious Beliefs?

	Under 35 Years	35-49 Years	50-64 Years	65+ Years
Extremely Important	76.29%	82.96%	79.56%	85.92%
Very Important	20.62%	16.08%	19.89%	12.68%
Fairly Important	3.09%	.96%	.55%	1.40%
Somewhat Important	0	0	0	0
Fairly Unimportant	0	0	0	0
Not at all Important	0	0	0	0
TOTAL	100%	100%	100%	100%

DOES SPIRITUALITY
INCREASE WITH AGE?

Analysis of data from a large 1994 national survey in the Lutheran Church-Missouri Synod similarly revealed that women aged sixty-five and over ranked highest on church attendance, personal prayer, importance of religious beliefs, biblical knowledge, serving others, personal faith, and other components of spirituality. However, this difference between age cohorts was not necessarily static, for the senior women also had increased more during as little as the previous two or three years than had the younger women on several measures of personal piety, God consciousness, and concern for others, as well as in their commitment to Jesus Christ and their sense of the importance of their spiritual lives (Moberg, 1999). As presented in Chapter 4, there are hints also from other research that as people age, their levels of spirituality are more likely to rise than fall, even though on the crude measures used in research to date the largest proportion show no obvious change at all.

Historical and personal life experiences may be responsible for the type and degree of religious identification of the aged. If we assume from Blazer and Palmore's (1976) longitudinal research that many people form their basic religious beliefs during their youth and also that there is increasing doubt among clergy and lay people regarding the central theological doctrines and relevancy of religious faith and practice, then it would follow that the aged should be more religious than younger persons (Rogers, 1976). This would also mean that elders have higher religiosity, take the Bible in a more literal sense than younger persons, possibly study the Bible more, and have a greater tendency to attend regular worship services.

Explanations of Age Differences

If the relationships between aging and spirituality are merely a reflection of cohort differences, then in a society that is increasingly secularized, we would expect each successive generation of aging people to become less religious and spiritual. Investigations for at least half a century, however, show a persistency that tends to reject that cohort hypothesis. Nevertheless, only longitudinal studies following large numbers of the same persons over time can settle the question of whether the aging process or cohort factors account for the age differences.

If it is true that people become more spiritual or religious with age, how can we account for that? Rogers (1976) claims that the universality of religion is based upon its social functions. He discusses four gerontological functions of religion:

1. To help face impending death.
2. To help find and maintain a sense of meaningfulness and significance in life.
3. To help accept the inevitable losses of old age and discover compensation values.
4. To meet secular social needs. (pp. 406-411)

In order to understand why people may become more spiritual or religious as they age, let us look at each of these functions. As people become older, their own impending demise becomes an ever more tangible possibility. This realization that one is not getting any younger can account for a tendency for religiosity to be integrated into life more as people age, specifically among people who were not particularly devout in their younger years. Herman J. Loether (1967) argues that this increase or tendency toward religiosity stems from one's fear of death. People tend to gravitate to religion in a search for comfort and an understanding of the impending end of human life.

A second gerontological function of aging is to help find and maintain a sense of meaningfulness and significance in life. Faith is nourished by the subjective need to face the anxiety of meaninglessness as finite humans facing the infinite mysteries of life and death. Religious goals provide compensation, most of all for those whose worldly lot seems intolerable. "There can be no 'rational' substitute for the belief that some unseen but benevolent force moves in mysterious ways to make man's fate meaningful and ultimately optimistic" (Hiltner, 1952, as quoted in Rogers, 1976, p. 408).

Martin Luther (1943) believed that man lives before God through faith, not good works, and because faith comes from what is heard, he emphasized the preaching of the Gospel rather than the performance of ritual acts. This "hearing" that leads to faith is the cornerstone upon which many of the aged are building to judge for themselves if their lives are meaningful and significant. They must sense a reason for existing. Again through the Gospel, God tells us that each life has a purpose. Everyone must have a source of strength to call upon, something that will help one to see one's life as meaningful. Otherwise no matter how well physical needs are met, one is likely to be unhappy and left without a sense of meaningfulness and or significance.

A third gerontological function of religion is to help accept the inevitable losses of old age and discover compensatory values. As individuals age, they begin to relinquish roles, especially through retirement. Even though this passage into retirement is planned and usually inevitable, the impact can be significant. This passing typically represents the loss of activities and often of a value structure upon which one's entire life was centered. Some use religion as a companion and comforter as they navigate their way through these transitions.

Barron (1961) claims that the Protestant religions generally have provided a basis for the formulation of numerous spiritual satisfactions that may serve as compensatory mechanisms in old age. These include:

1. Assurance of God's continuing love.
2. Certainty that life is protected.
3. Relief from heightened emotions as of fear, guilt, grief.
4. Relief from loneliness.
5. A perspective for life that embraces time and eternity.
6. Continued spiritual growth.
7. A satisfying status in life as a person.
8. The illusion of continued worth and usefulness. (p. 167)

The last gerontological function of religion Rogers (1976) lists is the meeting of secular social needs. Compared to other institutions, the church is in a unique position to provide spiritual support to aging people, but usually it can do that fully only as a by-product of meeting their more secular social needs. In order to carry out God's ministry effectively, it is imperative that church staff know these members by name and have a general understanding of their life circumstances. For example, do the persons reside in a nursing home, are they shut-ins, have they recently lost a loved one? This basic knowledge will help the church to understand what it is the aged need. Feeling like a part of the church community, the aged will be more comfortable and the church will then have created an environment to allow them to fulfill their secular social needs.

Hypotheses About Late-Life Religion

Although it is clear that religion has the capacity to satisfy many needs and that older people generally tend to be more spiritual than younger people, they may not attend church more. Orbach's (1961) analysis of 6,911 adults in the Detroit Metropolitan Area found that age as such was not related to differences in church attendance except for a decrease among those past age seventy-five. His findings led Rogers (1976) to the following hypotheses (generalizations to test in research) about why individuals may become more religious in late life.

Diminished Life Space and Opportunity

Religion allows an outlet for those over sixty to remain active by investing emotional energy and making a commitment that helps them to age with a purpose and grace.

Egocentric Defense

As people age, they are faced with the realization that they, their families and friends become afflicted with infirmities that contradict their youthfulness. Egocentric defense relates to religion based on the premise that as people age, their youthfulness eventually succumbs to old age and then to death. The finality of death, from which no mortal returns, brings wonderment and anxiety about the unknown afterlife. Therefore, one of the gerontological functions of religion is to help face impending death.

Decreased Mental Capacity

Studies show, say Pressey and Kuhlen (1957), that older people are more likely to have a tendency to be annoyed by minute wrongs, and they give more moralistic views about behavior. It seems that there is no middle ground; many of the elderly allegedly see things in black and white and make decisions on absolute moral bases. Because older people are not touched as intimately by social changes, their tendency to be more secluded could account for the age differences in values and differential religious identification.

Increased Tendency Toward Introspection

The self-examination of one's own life, whether through a formal or informal life review (see Chapter 12), can be a powerful persuader toward religious reform. When one examines the gerontological functions of religion, this can be closely associated with the quest to find meaningfulness and significance in life.

Putative and Punitive Control

Biological and social processes could heighten increased religiosity. This may contribute to an increased defensiveness and rigidity that account for the aged's tendency to accept social norms and conventional behavior without question, instead of exhibiting plasticity. Religion generally includes definitions of acceptable social behavior, and as a result it directs people to behave according to religious norms, such as the Ten Commandments, without questions. Rigid adherence to religious norms may be a method by which disengaged seniors attempt to exercise control after withdrawing from the active world.

Stereotype-Confirming Visibility

Since it is expected that aged people become more religious, their high degree of visibility and presence in religious functions may be more apparent.

Generational Differences

The aged may have been exposed to a belief system during their socialization process that is no longer among beliefs generally accepted. In other words, a cohort effect reflects doctrines prescribed during the socialization days of today's population over age sixty that are probably different from those accepted by today's youth.

To our knowledge, these seven hypotheses about changes in religiousness and spirituality have not been tested, although it is likely that clinicians, counselors, pastors, and others who serve elderly people have anecdotal evidence that bears upon them.

CONCLUSIONS AND IMPLICATIONS

Most research to date reveals higher levels of religiousness and spirituality among aging Americans than among young and middle-aged people. Echoing Gallup polls, the 1990 General Social Survey revealed that at least weekly religious attendance is more common among successively older cohorts of Americans and highest of all among those past age sixty-five (Levin, 1997). The main exception sometimes found is lower levels of participation in out-of-the-home religious activity among the old-old, many of whom suffer various forms of infirmity. But as discussed in Chapter 4, even when organizational forms of religiosity decrease, nonorganizational spirituality can remain high or even increase. Obviously, these complications offer rich opportunities for careful research.

Because religion, and especially spirituality, is so important to large numbers of older people, every possible effort should be made to incorporate spiritual needs into services in long-term care and religious communities. For example, it may prove beneficial to integrate into elementary and high school curriculums some activities that intermingle young and old people. This integration or mentoring will extend an opportunity to the aging community to maintain their meaningfulness, dignity, and significance in life, while also providing youth with a stable, concrete example of what life is all about. The younger generation would learn from their elders that people are given only one opportunity to live, so life should be lived as one's only chance to make a contribution. If the younger generation can see through the eyes of the aged that spiritual and other decisions made today will affect their lives tomorrow, this will prepare them to thoughtfully consider their options and choose those which will enhance their lives and the lives of those around them. If this outcome is achieved, we may see that the goal of increased spirituality and religiosity is not just for the aged alone.

Death faces everyone as an inevitable facet of the life experience. Religion tries to reconcile people to this destiny by giving it meaning in superempirical terms (Rogers, 1976). If the ultimate function of religion is to provide meaning for life and hope for life after death, an increase in the importance of religion in a person's life as one ages is logical. The Christian faith of the women in the Lutheran study offers hope for a life after death.

As a Christian, the most superempirical evidence we are given is the fact that Jesus died on the cross for our sins and rose again to reward all believers, with the ultimate gift, an eternal life with God. As believers our life's goal is to draw ever closer to the ultimate in religiosity and spirituality, the fulfillment of God's promise of a life after death with Him.

Undisputedly, death is an inevitable facet of the life experience. Nonetheless, the promises of the Bible assure believers, whether young or old, that God "will wipe every tear from their eyes. There will be no more death or mourning or crying or pain, for the old order of things has passed away" (Revelation 21:4, NIV). With a promise such as this, does it really matter if science can prove conclusively that religiosity and spirituality increase with age?

REFERENCES

Baker, David C. and Paul D. Nussbaum (1997). Religious practice and spiritual-ity—Then and now: A retrospective study of spiritual dimensions of residents resid-ing at a continuing care retirement community, *Journal of Religious Gerontology* 10(3):33-51.

Barna, George (1994). *Virtual America.* Ventura, CA: Regal Books.

Barron, Milton L. (1961). *The aging American: An introduction to social gerontology and geriatrics.* New York: Thomas Y. Crowell Co.

Bianchi, Eugene C. (1984). *Aging as a spiritual journey.* New York: Crossroad Pub-lishing Co.

Blazer, Dan and Erdman Palmore (1976). Religion and aging in a longitudinal panel. *The Gerontologist* 6:82-85.

Cavan, R. S., E.W. Burgess, R. J. Havighurst, and H. Goldhamer (1949). *Personal ad-justment in old age.* Chicago: Science Research Associates.

Fischer, Kathleen R. (1992). Spirituality and the aging family: A systems perspective. *Journal of Religious Gerontology* 8(4):1-15.

Hall, G.S. (1922). *Senescence: The second half of life.* New York: Appleton.

Hiltner, Seward (1952). Religion and the aging process. In *Notable papers on aging,* No. 5. New York: National Committee on Aging. Quoted in Tommy Rogers, Mani-festations of religiosity and the aging process. *Religious Education* 71(4):408, 1976.

Holmes, Urban T. (1982). *Spirituality for ministry.* San Francisco: Harper & Row.

Johnson, Ben C. (1989). Spirituality and the later years. *Journal of Religion and Aging* 6(3/4):125-139.

Jones, Paul W. (1984). Aging as a spiritualizing process. *Journal of Religion and Aging* 1(1):3-16.

Levin, Jeffrey S. (1997). Religious research in gerontology, 1980-1994: A systematic Review. *Journal of Religious Gerontology* 10(3):3-31.

Loether, Herman J. (1967). *Problems of aging: Sociological and social psychological perspectives.* Belmont, CA: Dickenson Publishing Company

Luther, Martin (1943). *A short explanation of Dr. Martin Luther's Small Cate-chism.* St. Louis, MO: Concordia Publishing House.

Moberg, David O. (1990). Spiritual maturity and wholeness in later years. *Journal of Religious Gerontology* 7(1/2):5-24.

Moberg, David O. (1997). Religion and aging. In Ferraro, Kenneth F. (Ed.), *Gerontol-ogy: Perspectives and issues,* Second edition (pp. 193-220). New York: Springer Publishing Company.

Moberg, David O. (1999). *Women of God: An assessment of the spirituality of women in the Lutheran Church-Missouri Synod.* St. Louis, MO: Lutheran Women's Mis-sionary League.

Niebuhr, H. Richard (1967). *The meaning of revelation.* New York: Macmillan.

NIV: *The Holy Bible,* New International Version (1984). Colorado Springs, CO: International Bible Society.

Orbach, Harold L. (1961). Aging and religion: A study of church attendance in the Detroit Metropolitan Area. *Geriatrics* 16(10):530-540.

Palmore, Erdman (1980). The social factors in aging. In Busse, E. and Dan Blazer (Eds.), *Handbook of geriatric psychiatry.* New York: Van Nostrand Reinhold.

Pressey, S. L. and R. G. Kuhlen (1957). *Psychological development through the life span.* New York: Harper and Brothers.

Rogers, Tommy (1976). Manifestations of religiosity and the aging process. *Religious Education* 71(4):405-415.

Starbuck, E. D. (1911). *The psychology of religion: An empirical study of the growth of religious consciousness.* New York: Walter Scott.

Stokes, Kenneth (1990). Faith development in the adult life cycle. In Seeber, James J. (Ed.), *Spiritual maturity in the later years* (pp. 167-184). Binghamton, NY: The Haworth Press.

PROFESSIONAL AND PRACTICAL APPLICATIONS

Today every agency, institution, and human service professional desiring to meet the full scope of human needs must give attention to spirituality. The next seven chapters provide examples of how this is being done in representative contexts, including health care, hospices, counseling, social work, and chaplaincies, each of which suggests possible replications and adaptations elsewhere.

On a more personal level, we shall see how "The Canticle of Brother Sun" by St. Francis of Assisi can be a tool for meditation and self-refection to stimulate anyone's spiritual growth. Another effective tool is the spiritual life review, which can be used by individuals alone, in their activities as members of either religious or secular groups, or as a part of clinical services. It helps people deal realistically with spiritual issues related to their past, present, and future.

People from every walk of life will benefit from these chapters. They provide suggestions and hints on how to help others spiritually, resources to aid volunteer and professional service activities, and clues for cultivating one's personal spirituality.

Chapter 7

Spiritual Care by Primary Health Care Providers

Allison E. Soerens

Over the past century, scientific and technological advances in the field of medicine have caused many health care providers to lose sight of the individual patients they are treating. In most cases, these professionals believe that health is merely the absence of disease. This simplistic view of health significantly impairs quality patient care by not recognizing that humans are multidimensional holistic beings. Borins (1984) asserts that the word "holistic" reemerged in the 1970s. It comes from the Greek word *holos,* meaning all encompassing. Those who view health as a positive sense of well-being or state of wholeness not only care for peoples' physical needs, but for their psychological, emotional, social, and spiritual needs as well. Health care providers who genuinely provide holistic health care incorporate spiritual care into their practice. Understanding the essence of spirituality and the implications it has for an individual's health is critical to providing high-quality health care.

While some primary health care providers believe the notion that spirituality or religious involvement positively influences health and clinical outcomes is inconceivable, others are beginning to recognize the invaluable benefits of spiritual care on patients' health. Both past and current research on the role of spirituality in health care has yielded supportive evidence of the positive influence of religion and spirituality on health. However, in the current fast-paced, cost-driven, high-tech health care environment, the significance of spirituality has been lost (Dyson, Cobb, and Forman, 1997). In addition, the lack of agreement on the definition and meaning of spirituality continues to impede progress in this area.

THE MEANING OF SPIRITUALITY

The definitions of spirituality are very diverse, yet arriving at a general consensus on the definition of spirituality is essential for research. Meaning and purpose in life, belief, and hope are universal hallmarks of human spirituality (Catterall et al., 1998). It is important to recognize that religious involvement is often a component of spirituality, but spirituality does not necessarily imply that a religious component is present. The ability to generalize research findings between these concepts is still being established. Catterall and colleagues (1998) define spirituality as "the lived experiences that give meaning to life and death" (p. 163). Lane (1987) further states, "The human spirit is a fragile vessel holding the essence of who we are" (p. 332). Moberg (1997) supports this statement. He gives further insight into the meaning of spirituality by stating, "One's spirit inevitably is implicated in everything we believe, do, and think, not in only a fraction of our behavior and thoughts" (as quoted by Ellor, 1997, p. 2).

RESEARCH ON SPIRITUALITY AND HEALTH

Prior to discussing the positive influence spirituality has on health, it is important to note that critics in the mental health field such as Sigmund Freud, Albert Ellis, and Wendall Waters have boldly claimed that religiosity negatively influences health. However, religion is only one component of spirituality, and research in this area has not supported their negative claims. Their accusations appear to be mere opinions with little substantiating evidence. In fact, Koenig (1997) in response reviewed numerous research studies and found that they indicate the positive effect of religiosity on health. For example, he found that four out of ten patients admitted to a tertiary-care teaching hospital believed religion was the most important factor that enabled them to cope. In addition, individuals with a higher degree of spiritual well-being and religious involvement were less likely to be treated for depression, anxiety, and alcohol or drug abuse.

According to Levin, Larson, and Puchalski (1997), research has shown that spirituality positively influences a person's ability to cope, decision to participate in health promoting behaviors, degree of supportive networks, and overall sense of well-being. Spiritual well-being enhances one's inner strength (Burkhardt, 1989). According to Conco (1995), research supports the fact that those who are spiritually well have a higher sense of well-being than those who are not, regardless of the presence of acute or chronic illness. Studies have further shown that individuals who regularly nurture their spirituality through religious practices, compared to those who do not, have a lower incidence of high blood pressure, heightened ability to cope with depression, decreased use of hospital services, and healthier immune systems (Mitka, 1998).

Catterall and colleagues (1998) found that many patients cite spiritual care as a dimension that enhances their well-being. Conco (1995) conducted a qualitative research study to assess the nature of spiritual care patients received during hospitalization. She interviewed three men and seven women ranging from age thirty-five to eighty-six who had been hospitalized for varying illnesses. The participants identified spiritual caregivers as ministers, nurses, doctors, family, friends, and nonprofessional hospital personnel. They believed their ability to cope with illness and recover was directly influenced by spiritual care, and they identified decreased anxiety, increased comfort, hope, inner strength, acceptance, optimism, and well-being as positive outcomes of spiritual care. Research conducted by Clark and colleagues (1991) supports these findings. They found that the most significant contributions to recovery perceived by recently hospitalized patients were support and hope.

Brooke (1987) states that it is the spiritual dimension that enables older adults to find meaning in their lives and cope with age-related problems. Berggren-Thomas and Griggs (1995) found that one way older adults nurture their spirituality is through church attendance. They determined that the benefits of church attendance include social interaction, emotional support, enhanced self-esteem, and spiritual growth. The studies in Seeber (1990) also support the notion that spiritual well-being is critical to successful aging.

Conversely, Kazanjian (1997) found that patients who perceive themselves as alone and helpless respond to age-related problems and serious and terminal health conditions with confusion and despair. In addition, Mor, McHorney, and Sherwood (1986) found that bereaved individuals seek medical care more frequently, but are no more likely to be hospitalized. They suggest that this health-seeking behavior is an attempt to gain social support. Perhaps this hypothesis can be expanded to state that these individuals are seeking spiritual support. Dyson, Cobb, and Forman (1997) suggest that in order to be truly happy and at peace one must have a sense of purpose and meaning in one's life. Illness, suffering, and death challenge personal meaning. Health care providers who care for their patients' spirituality assist them in developing effective coping skills and finding meaning in their life experiences.

This body of research illustrates the positive links between spirituality and health. Furthermore, it supports the hypothesis that the integration of spiritual care into therapy by primary health care providers enhances the quality of care patients receive. However, despite the vast body of evidence supporting the correlation between spirituality and positive health outcomes, spiritual care is still an underutilized therapy modality by health care providers.

CURRENT PRACTICE

The nursing community has been known for its commitment to providing holistic patient care, of which spiritual care is a necessary component. David B. Larson, MD, president of the National Institute for Health Care Research, believes that physicians are ready to integrate spiritual care into their practices, providing there is adequate scientific research to support its use (Mitka, 1998). Primary health care providers are in an excellent position to integrate the spiritual with the physical and psychosocial, providing true holistic care. For many individuals, religious beliefs and practices are an essential component of their spirituality.

Maugans and Wadland (1991) interviewed 115 physicians in primary health care and 135 patients whom they cared for, to investigate the perceived role of religion in health care. They found that actual inquiry regarding the religious beliefs and practices of a patient was infrequent. The most reported opportunity to address these issues by both patients and physicians was in the context of a serious or life-threatening event. However, 30 percent of both groups also recognized health care maintenance visits as an acceptable time to assess religiosity. Two barriers to providing spiritual care identified by this study were a lack of formal training and a belief that it is primarily the patient's responsibility to address religious issues. However, over 40 percent of the patients welcomed physician inquiry about spiritual and religious matters. Greene and colleagues (1987) support this finding. They concluded that patients do respond favorably to physician-initiated inquiries regarding spiritual well-being.

BELIEFS ABOUT PROVIDING SPIRITUAL CARE

The author conducted an exploratory, qualitative, research study to assess primary health care provider students' attitudes and beliefs regarding spiritual care. A seven-item interview guide with open-ended questions concerning spiritual care was designed for this purpose. The following questions were utilized during the interview process:

- How do you define spirituality?
- Do you feel you have sufficient skills and knowledge to nurture patients' spirituality?
- Have you received any formal training on spiritual care? If so, was it through a required or elective class?
- How can a primary health care provider give spiritual care to patients?
- How often do you participate in this type of care?
- What are the barriers, if any, to providing spiritual care?
- Do you believe spirituality has a role in the delivery of health care by primary care providers? Explain your answer.

A convenience sample of ten nurse practitioner and medical students were interviewed. Confidentiality of the respondents was assured. Consent was implied by completion of the interview.

Participants defined spirituality as a person's connection to a purpose or calling; faith in a higher being; sense of purpose in life, meaning, value, and direction; an inner connection with one's soul; a relationship with God; and a belief system that helps a person find one's inner self. When asked if they had received any formal training on spiritual care, 50 percent responded "no," while only 10 percent stated they had received education regarding spiritual care through a required course. Furthermore, 60 percent of the respondents stated that they did not feel they had sufficient skills and knowledge to nurture a patient's spirituality. However, they unanimously believed spirituality had a role in the delivery of health care by primary health care providers. In addition, they identified a variety of interventions that primary care providers can implement to enhance their patients' spirituality. These included listening, being present, giving positive feedback, offering a supportive attitude, facilitating expression, exploring spiritual resources, being aware of one's own spirituality, providing holistic assessment, conveying an interest and willingness to discuss spiritual matters, offering support of religious personnel, and praying with patients. Barriers to giving spiritual care were perceived as a lack of time, limited knowledge base, lack of rapport, environmental constraints, and patients' unwillingness to discuss spiritual matters.

Due to small size, the findings of the study cannot be generalized to a larger population, although they have several implications. This study implies that there is a lack of education regarding spiritual care of patients in academic health care study. As is evident here and in Chapter 4, research supports the positive effects of spirituality on health. Clearly, it is an integral part of holistic health care. Future investigation of primary health care provider curricula is necessary. In addition, although half of the respondents did not believe they were equipped to provide spiritual care, all were able to identify spiritual care interventions. This suggests that, although advanced course work, seminars, and workshops heighten an individual's knowledge and ability to give spiritual care, many individuals, as spiritual beings, intuitively know how to nurture the spiritual realm. Finally, time was the most frequently reported barrier to giving spiritual care. Future research utilizing indicators that genuinely reflect spiritual care outcomes must be performed in order to justify time spent on spiritual care and subsequent reimbursement for those services by primary health care providers.

SPIRITUAL CARE INTERVENTIONS

Clark and colleagues (1991) assert that "quality care must enable holistic integration of the patient's inner resources" (p. 68). Spirituality is an integral part of holistic care. Coughlin (1996) states that "honoring spirituality means respecting another's journey and walking with them" (p. 65). Dyson, Cobb, and Forman (1997) suggest that both religious and nonreligious belief systems be considered in the exploration of spirituality and that spirituality should not be approached with embarrassment or hesitation.

Primary health care providers need to be sensitive to patients' spiritual needs. The more vulnerable a patient or family, the more spiritual care is required. In order to implement appropriate interventions, an accurate assessment of the spiritual resources of patients, and of their families when applicable, is essential (Kazanjian, 1997). Establishing a trusting relationship and supportive environment is necessary for accurate spiritual assessment (Clark et al., 1991).

Primary health care providers are able to offer patients numerous spiritual care interventions. For example, actively listening to a patient's feelings, whether positive or negative, honors spirituality. Discussing patients' religious affiliations, spiritual rituals, attitudes, beliefs, and relationships with others honors their spirituality (Coughlin, 1996). All of these domains are personal resources. Health care providers need to recognize spiritual strength and need to vary between patients and specific situations. Patients need to be allowed to share their thoughts, dreams, and memories. Prayer can further strengthen patients' spiritual networks. In addition, spiritual care includes health care providers sharing their own experiences of discovering meaning and purpose and their acceptance of and availability to their patient who is seeking meaning and purpose. Being present, taking time, touching, maintaining belief, enabling, and listening are all among the behaviors that nurture spiritual care (Conco, 1995).

Mitka (1998) suggests that patients' spirituality be assessed in an early visit. It should be done before a serious or terminal disease is diagnosed. In addition, when a patient is diagnosed with a chronic or terminal disease, it is imperative that the patient be given the opportunity to discuss what the diagnosis means to them and how they perceive their own future. "Research has shown that patients respond best to physician-initiated inquiries" (Maugans and Wadland, 1991, p. 212). Borins (1995) also suggests that an appointment immediately following a loss enables health care providers to assess their patients' spiritual needs and gives patients the opportunity to cry and express the meaning of their loss.

Providers need to be empathetic and genuine. Borins (1995) has found that patients in spiritual distress often invent physical symptoms as a way to get their foot in the door if they believe it is inappropriate to discuss spiritual matters with their health care provider. When this occurs, he suggests managing the acute situation and scheduling a follow-up appointment specifically to discuss spiritual needs. Primary health care providers need to be knowledgeable about community support groups and spiritual leaders that are able to offer further spiritual care.

In recent years, the term "life review" has become a buzzword, especially in hospice and nursing home settings. The life review is a phenomenological approach to or constructive retrospection of one's life (see Chapter 12). Hateley (1985) gives practical suggestions on how to assist patients with this process and discusses the many positive benefits this intervention yields. A spiritual life review creates the opportunity for those individuals involved to integrate their personality, draw conclusions about both the negative and positive aspects of their lives, find meaning in their existence, and direct their future life journey.

CURRICULUM AND SPIRITUAL CARE

Although there are multiple interventions that primary care providers can implement to nurture patients' spirituality, these interventions are underutilized. One reason for this is the lack of educational content on spirituality and health. Spirituality is often superficially addressed or subsumed under psychological care in the health care curriculum (Narayanasamy, 1993). Most schools in the United States do an excellent job of teaching primary care providers how to care for patients' physical needs; however, patients' psychosocial, emotional, and spiritual needs are often not adequately addressed. Fortunately, over the last fifteen years a growing emphasis on prevention and wellness has emerged. Providing holistic care has become an integral component to this approach.

As stated earlier, nursing has traditionally embraced holistic care, caring for patients' psychosocial, emotional, and spiritual needs as well as their physical needs. However, it is evident by the qualitative study conducted by this author and by this review of nursing literature that there is need for a more comprehensive education regarding the spiritual care of patients. Many nursing schools have recognized this need and have improved their curricula by expanding the religious and spiritual content offered at both the undergraduate and graduate level. In addition, according to Levin, Larson, and Puchalski (1997), the number of medical schools in the United States offering courses on religious and spiritual care has increased tenfold in the last few years.

FUTURE CONCERNS

Spiritual care can no longer be left to pastors and a few others designated as spiritual leaders. It should not be viewed as separate from other health care needs of patients, but seen rather as an integral part of patients' overall care (Catterall et al., 1998). Spiritual care by primary health care providers is a responsibility, not an option. "Integral to a more humanistic educational approach is enhancing students' receptivity when patients wish to talk about beliefs which give their lives meaning" (Levin, Larson, and Puchalski, 1997, p. 792).

Primary health care providers need to be comfortable with their own spirituality. Coughlin (1996) states, "Honoring our spirituality means strengthening our awareness of our spirit by paying attention with response and deep concentration to the spiritual qualities within ourselves and one another" (p. 65). Self-awareness and sensitivity teaching is critical to enabling health care providers to care adequately for patients' spiritual needs (Ross, 1997). The more aware we are of our own spirituality, the better equipped we are to nurture others on their spiritual journey.

Required rather than merely elective courses on religion and spirituality are suggested. Courses that review research on health, religion, and spirituality and teach practitioners how to assess, develop, and incorporate patients' spirituality into their health care are imperative. Competent spiritual care through innovative didactic and clinical training must be incorporated into both nursing and medical school curriculums. In addition, workshops geared for primary health care providers need to be offered to enhance the practitioners' ability to effectively deliver spiritual care.

Future investigations in the areas of spiritual assessment instruments, barriers to spiritual care, and the direct and indirect effects of spiritual nurture on patient health need to be conducted (Maugans and Wadland, 1991). Spiritual assessment tools that are easy to follow and understand regardless of age or culture are needed. Because not all patients are religious, spiritual assessment tools that are free from religious bias are necessary. Borins (1984) states, "The more tools we have for dealing with the many problems that do not respond to drugs and surgery, the better medicine will be able to confront the challenges of the next century" (p. 105).

Finally, barriers to spiritual care are often attributed to time constraints. This factor can no longer be accepted. Clearly, the research illustrates a strong positive link between spirituality and health. Spiritual care must therefore be viewed as an integral component of primary health care. Future research utilizing indicators that genuinely reflect spiritual care outcomes must be performed to determine effectiveness and to justify the time spent on spiritual care and the subsequent reimbursement for those services given by primary health care providers. Consequently, documentation of spiritual assessment and interventions must be thorough to illustrate these outcomes. Furthermore, large cross-sectional research studies are needed to improve the generalizability of the findings.

REFERENCES

Berggren-Thomas, P. and M. J. Griggs (1995). Spirituality in aging. Spiritual need or spiritual journey? *Journal of Gerontological Nursing* 21(3):5-10.

Borins, M. (1984). Holistic medicine in family practice. *Canadian Family Physician* 30:101-106.

Borins, M. (1995). Grief counseling. *Canadian Family Physician* 41:1207-1211.

Brooke, V. (1987). The spiritual well-being of the elderly. *Geriatric Nursing* 8(4): 194-195.

Burkhardt, M. (1989). Spirituality: An analysis of the concept. *Holistic Nursing Practice* 3(3):69-77.

Catterall, R. A., M. Cox, B. Greet, J. Sankey, and G. Griffiths (1998). Spiritual care: The assessment and audit of spiritual care. *International Journal of Palliative Nursing* 4(4):162-168.

Clark, C. C., J. R. Cross, D. M. Deane, and L. W. Lowry (1991). Spirituality: Integral to quality care. *Holistic Nursing Practice* 5(3):67-76.

Conco, D. (1995). Christian patients' views of spiritual care. *Journal of Nursing Research* 17(3):266-276.

Coughlin, D. M. (1996). Honoring the spirituality of grieving parents. *Home Care Provider* 1(2):63-67.

Dyson, J., M. Cobb, and D. Forman (1997). The meaning of spirituality: A literature review. *Journal of Advanced Nursing* 26(6):1183-1188.

Ellor, J. W. (1997). Spiritual well-being defined. *Aging & Spirituality* 9(1):1-2.

Greene, M. G., S. Hoffman, R. Charon, and R. Adelman (1987). Psychosocial concerns in the medical encounter: A comparison of doctors' interactions with their old and young patients. *Gerontologist* 27(2):164-168.

Hateley, B. J. (1985). *Telling your story, exploring your faith: Writing your life history for personal insight and spiritual growth.* St Louis, MO: CBD Press.

Kazanjian, M. A. (1997). The spiritual and psychological explanations for loss experience. *The Hospice Journal* 12(1):17-27.

Koenig, H. G. (1997). *Is religion good for your health? The effects of religion on physical and mental health.* Binghamton, New York: The Haworth Press.

Lane, J. A. (1987). Care of the human spirit. *Journal of Professional Nursing* 3(16): 332-337.

Levin, J. S., D. B. Larson, and C. M. Puchalski (1997). Religion and spirituality in medicine: Research and education. *Journal of the American Medical Association* 278(9): 792-793.

Maugans, T. A. and W. C. Wadland (1991). Religion and family medicine: A survey of physicians and patients. *The Journal of Family Practice* 32(2):210-213.

Mitka, M. (1998). Getting religion seen as help in being well. *Journal of the American Medical Association* 280(22):1896-1897.

Moberg, D. O. (1997). Spiritual well-being defined: A response. *Aging & Spirituality* 9(1):8.

Mor, V., C. McHorney, and S. Sherwood (1986). Secondary morbidity among the recently bereaved. *American Journal of Psychiatry* 143(2):158-163.

Narayanasamy, A. (1993). Nurses' awareness and educational preparation in meeting their patients' spiritual needs. *Nurse Education Today* 13(3):196-201.

Ross, L. (1997). The nurse's role in assessing and responding to patients' spiritual needs. *International Journal of Palliative Nursing* 3(1):37-42.

Seeber, J. J. (Ed.) (1990). *Spiritual maturity in the later years.* Binghamton, New York: The Haworth Press.

Chapter 8

Spiritual Care in Hospice Settings

Edith Anne Glascock Angeli

Hospice care can be defined as providing palliative, as opposed to curative, care for dying patients with a prognosis of six months or less. The care received can vary between patients; however, it is usually limited to comfort measures such as pain management. Although hospices provide care for patients facing the end of their life, they support and maintain the importance of providing wholistic care until the last moment of the patient's life, and beyond. Great strides have been made to address ways to care for the mind and body. The spirit, however, has been left behind in the fast-paced environment of health care.

This chapter provides an understanding of how a layperson can provide spiritual care for the diverse population of hospice patients. First, the analysis process includes studying the role of spiritual care in a hospice environment and examining questions and concerns facing hospice patients that are unique to those suffering from a terminal illness. Many of those concerns are related to the spiritual self, for which caregivers are often asked to provide support and guidance.

Another important process in moving toward an understanding of spiritual care is summarizing the views expressed by hospice caregivers. Both spiritual and hospice care are relatively new to the United States. New philosophies and practices bring questions of how, when, and by whom the care should be provided.

Next, included in this analysis is a summary and evaluation of results from a national survey on spiritual care and the dying process. Its findings provide insights into what Americans consider truly important in spiritual care and the part caregivers play in meeting a patient's spiritual needs. Finally, a summary of personal conclusions is provided.

UNDERSTANDING
THE HOSPICE PHILOSOPHY

The philosophy of hospice care was developed in London, England, after World War II by Dame Cicely Saunders, MD (Flood, 1984). In 1975, the first hospice in the United States was opened in New Haven, Connecticut. Its new philosophy confronted deeply held social taboos about death and such terminal illnesses as cancer, heart disease, and, more recently, AIDS.

Today, there are approximately 2,500 hospices serving people in every state of the United States. Dame Saunders summed up the hospice philosophy best when she stated, "You matter to the last moment of your life, and we will do all we can, not only to help you die peacefully, but to live until you die" (NHO, 1996). Hospice care supports the belief that health care should treat the mind, body, and spirit. To provide this type of wholistic approach, a team of social workers, nurses, and spiritual counselors are involved with creating a care plan for each patient.

Hospice philosophy has four principal components. The first is that physical care is primarily the palliation of the pain and discomfort associated with terminal illness. Second, hospice care includes refraining from intervention by means of CPR or other life-saving techniques when a patient's heart stops or respiration ceases. Third, emotional support is provided by all members of the hospice team for the patient and family, including bereavement counseling. Finally, spiritual needs were originally addressed by arranging assistance from a minister, priest, or rabbi for the patient and family. Views on spiritual care, however, have evolved.

That evolution is partially due to efforts made by hospice care providers to expand their own understanding of the role that spiritual care plays in the last days of a terminal patient's life. Those efforts include attempts to define spirituality and to evaluate the importance of spiritual care to the overall comfort of each hospice patient. Gaining some understanding of spirituality and spiritual care will help every individual responsible for providing care for terminally ill patients.

DEFINING SPIRITUALITY AND SPIRITUAL CARE

Defining spirituality and spiritual care is a study in and of itself. One major obstacle in addressing spirituality is that all human beings have individual belief and value systems that influence their understanding of these terms. Philosophers, psychologists, and theologians have speculated endlessly about what it means to be human and about the nature and interaction of mind, body, and spirit. Despite the complexity of the arguments, we humans are both body and spirit; we face life in ways that are more than physical reactions, and our understanding of what it means to be human includes a dimension that both encompasses and goes beyond our physicality.

Sheehan (1997) offers this definition of spirituality:

> There are at least three components to this spiritual dimension. First, spirituality is an expression of how a person relates to a larger whole, be it God, a higher power, or the human family. Second, personal spirituality provides a source of meaning and understanding about the significance of being human. Third, personal spirituality often contains habits, rituals, gestures, and symbols that provide ways in which the person can interpret and manage existence. (p. 1)

For the purpose of this chapter, spirituality and religion are not synonymous. I assume that Sheehan's definition encompasses the idea that a person can be spiritual without explicit religious beliefs or practices. Spirituality helps individuals find meaning in life and understand their behaviors and the choices they make. The spirituality of a person develops and grows with age, and it remains important (if not more so) when one is facing death.

Some health care professionals become nervous when asked about the role of spirituality in medicine. Many assume that spiritual care requires enforcing particular religious beliefs (Carr, 1995). Religious beliefs indeed are one way in which people can express their spirituality. However, it cannot be assumed that each person subscribes to a particular religion, nor that religion is the main focus of someone who is facing the end of life. Spiritual beliefs and religious values are not the same. Nonreligious values and meanings in life are sometimes called spiritual, and spiritual pain often is very deep (Kearney, 1990). Therefore, spiritual assessments must include a broader evaluation of a person's values and interiorized creed than one that is limited to his or her religion.

Kearney understands these as the essence of being human. They include issues about the soul, the self, values, and the meaning in life. Such values are not dependent on a particular religion, but are a part of every human being throughout life, without regard to one's religiosity. Caregivers are faced with treating many different individuals with varying illnesses and varying needs. Some of those needs may center around the patient's spirituality.

In a hospice setting, assessing physical needs has similarities from patient to patient. The main goal is to alleviate pain and assist patients to make them as comfortable as possible. As physical abilities diminish, hospice caregivers look for alternate ways to care for patients. For example, some patients who develop difficulties in swallowing food are provided with pureed food or a liquid diet. Another example is the use of a catheter when a patient becomes incontinent. Treating physical symptoms is somewhat easier because they are usually visible and/or more obvious to the caregiver. Spiritual needs can be elusive to the patient, not to mention the caregiver.

Most hospice facilities have developed their own spiritual-needs assessments for patients and families. For example, Milwaukee Hospice Homecare and Residence has created an assessment to identify and evaluate spiritual care needs that is often done prior to the patient's entering hospice care. The completed form is available to caregivers at all times, so a continuous assessment is possible. Although its questions provide some assistance and direction for caregivers, they still may not open the door for the patient to discuss spiritual feelings and questions. One way to improve the usefulness of this type of assessment is to provide spiritual care training for caregivers.

The training of volunteers at Milwaukee Hospice focuses largely on ways to communicate effectively with terminal patients. This type of training is essential to preparing someone for the unique environment of hospice care. However, the training for spiritual care can be summed up in this way: Make efforts to contact the patient's religious counselor or to inform one of the hospice directors if a patient is requesting spiritual guidance or care. In reality, however, hospice caregivers are often treating spiritual needs without realizing they are doing so (Kearney, 1990).

The Importance of Spiritual Care

Why is spiritual care such an integral part of hospice care? The original reason that spiritual care became a part of the modern hospice movement is because pioneers like Dame Saunders saw the importance of caring for the whole person (wholistic care—mind, body, and spirit) during the dying process. Three considerations support the importance of spiritual care.

The first reason a hospice team should be concerned with spiritual care is that acknowledging and inquiring about a patient's spirituality provides a deeper insight into the patient's experience (Sheehan, 1997). Hospice caregivers participate in one of the most significant aspects of human life, the dying process. They are confronted with and can share in their patients' feelings of hope, despair, joy, and profound sorrow. Patients can remain in hospice care for as little as a few days to as long as a few months. Provided their physician's prognosis for their survival is six months or less, the patient is eligible for funding of this type of care under Medicare or health insurance. If the hospice team is fortunate, its members will have the opportunity to spend time getting to know their patient and perhaps to learn a little more about what made this person unique.

Second, getting to know more chapters of a patient's life, including gaining insight into his or her spiritual journey, can provide a context for making decisions in planning care (Sheehan, 1997). Although almost all care decisions are made upon the patient's entrance into a hospice, due to the nature of the care (i.e., there will be no use of extraordinary means to prolong life), the patient and family will still face decisions related to emotional and spiritual care. Caregivers may want to allow for additional support by arranging for a volunteer to sit with the patient or to spend increased time addressing any fears and concerns expressed by the patient.

A third reason hospice caregivers should be concerned with a patient's spiritual needs is that it can allow caregivers to help patients in a way that is fundamental to hospice care: limiting suffering and not abandoning the patient during the experiences of illness and death (Kearney, 1990). As people die, they could be in spiritual distress as deep as any physical pain. Allowing a patient to express spiritual pain is one way to help heal a person's spirit, especially when physical healing is no longer possible (Sheehan, 1997). It is beneficial to the care of hospice patients if their caregivers are open to addressing their spiritual needs or are willing to help them find spiritual resources (e.g., books, music, a clergyperson, etc.).

In addition, many end-of-life decisions typically are deferred until death is imminent and anxieties run high. Helping patients and their families cope with these is another important contribution of hospice care (Munly, 1983).

PROVIDING SPIRITUAL CARE FOR HOSPICE PATIENTS

The role that spiritual care plays in a hospice setting has been considered. How, then, do hospice caregivers provide spiritual support and care for those in need? One characteristic often associated with hospice patients is a sense of urgency. The amount of time remaining for each patient is uncertain, so he or she is usually conservative with how time is spent. One of the greatest gifts a patient can give to a caregiver is sharing intimately personal thoughts and feelings. However, he or she needs to be prepared if the patient is unintentionally or unconsciously searching for support and guidance in addressing spiritual needs.

Initially, providing spiritual care could be interpreted simply as praying with the patient, reading Scriptures, or performing some other type of religious practice or ritual. These narrow interpretations, however, could impose barriers between caregivers and their patients.

One of the most repeated opinions in available therapy is that spiritual care must be provided without bias or concern for the provider's personal beliefs. The role of spiritual care in a hospice should not influence the beliefs of others or force answers to questions that engulf the waking hours of the terminally ill (Carr, 1995). Because spirituality is often associated with religion, it is natural to look to one's own religious beliefs as a template for relating to others. With an expanded understanding of spirituality, caregivers and patients may find comfort in knowing that spiritual care is not limited by the boundaries of organized religion.

An essential characteristic of being a caregiver in a hospice setting is to be comfortable with holding a stranger's hand and sitting in silence without feeling the need to speak. These simple actions can provide the environment a patient needs to feel a sense of security and serenity. Some believe that creating this kind of environment is one example of providing spiritual care. Simply being available to listen without judgment can allow a patient to reflect on inner feelings and concerns, even if those feelings and concerns are not verbalized. Patients who choose to share their questions or fears will most likely be comforted by the fact that the caregiver will listen with open ears, an open mind, and a closed mouth.

One question that is often asked by terminally ill patients is "Why?" Questions such as "Why me?" and "Why now?" are indicators of spiritual pain (Carr, 1995). The feelings often expressed are fear, despair, guilt, failure, and hopelessness. Once these signs emerge, those who are caring for the dying can help the patient recognize what is going on and let the patient find meaning in this distress. Such instances of listening on the part of the caregiver can bring about some spiritual peace and quiet for the patient that Kearney (1990) describes as experiences of connection, alignment, harmony, and meaningfulness. Ultimately, it is the patient who knows which resolutions help to relieve spiritual pain.

Kearney also believes that spiritual peace and healing can just happen on their own. Even though those who care for hospice patients can help in the spiritual-healing process, it is the dying who heal themselves. He reminds us that no one can provide absolute answers for the dying; our own "personal answers" about life and death should not be imposed upon someone else in an attempt to heal spiritual pain. This supports the importance of having caregivers listen to their patients. One of Kearney's main theories is that those caring for terminally ill patients should simply enable their patients to determine their meaning and win back or achieve spiritual peace.

Another consideration for hospice caregivers is that, similar to other aspects of the dying process, spiritual health and well-being can have different meanings for each individual patient. For some, spiritual peace may come from the patient's turning his or her life over to Jesus Christ. For others, however, spiritual peace may come from addressing unresolved issues with family or loved ones or from reliving their life's contributions through stories and photographs. It is not uncommon that, during their final journey, hospice patients find comfort by searching for the positive effects their life had on the world around them (Saunders, 1975).

Hospice care was originally intended to provide a period of rest for loved ones who were caring for a terminally ill patient. A hospice care provider would come into the home of the patient to relieve some of the pressure on the caregivers (e.g., through performing personal services for the patient, assisting with household chores, etc.). The intention was to allow the primary caregiver an opportunity to spend quality time with loved ones. With the creation of hospice facilities, family and friends have even more time to spend with the dying patient. This generally is seen as a positive aspect of hospice care. What also can happen, though, is that family and friends then witness more of the spiritual and emotional distress felt by the patient.

Sometimes the distress felt by the terminally ill patient manifests itself through obsessive-compulsive acts. These can include organizing and reorganizing personal effects or writing and rewriting lists. Witnessing such distress felt by a loved one can be very difficult, especially since there is no immediate or clear-cut remedy. Suffering, anguish, and confusion are often signs of spiritual pain (Sheehan, 1997). Dame Saunders (1975) saw spiritual pain as one part of the "total pain" felt by the dying; it is also the part that can be the most difficult to define. A patient's loved ones may find some comfort in understanding what might be the cause of the patient's behavior changes, even if little can be done to reduce the spiritual distress.

One obstacle standing in the way of gaining a better understanding of spirituality in hospice care is associated with assessing the care provided for a terminally ill patient. One characteristic inherent in the hospice philosophy is the cessation of invasive treatment. It can be argued that asking hospice patients to "rate" any of the care they receive is invading their time for self-reflection and moving the focus from the patient to the institution. However, a national survey has been done in an attempt to better understand spiritual care; more specifically, to explore spiritual beliefs and how they relate to the dying process.

A POLL ON SPIRITUAL BELIEFS
AND DYING

In October 1997, the George H. Gallup International Institute published results from a national survey of spiritual beliefs and the dying process. This study asked people to look into the future that lies ahead for every human being, and describe what kind of care they would like to receive during their dying days (see Table 8.1).

This survey of 1,212 adults (over the age of eighteen) provides specific guidance to those who have a concern or responsibility for persons who are actively dying—family and friends, physicians, other medical people, clergy and other religious counselors, social workers, and volunteers, to name a few. The results demonstrate that any person who is involved in caring for a terminally ill patient can also play a part in providing spiritual care and that the American people want to reassert the spiritual dimension of care for the dying.

Table 8.1. Types of Comforting Support Desired When Dying, by Gender and Race/Ethnicity

			Gender		Race/Ethnicity	
Type of Support	All (1,212) %	Male (481) %	Female (731) %	White (971) %	Minority (226) %
Having someone with whom you can share your fears or concerns	55	45	65	54	62
Having someone with you	54	43	63	54	55
Having someone holding your hand or touching you	47	37	56	48	47
Having someone help you to become spiritually at peace	44	35	53	42	54
Having someone pray with you	44	36	51	43	51
Having someone read spiritual or inspirational materials	32	26	37	28	48
Having someone perform ritual prayers or liturgies	21	19	23	18	32
Having someone read to you, other than religious materials	13	10	16	11	21

Source: Nathan Cummings Foundation, 1998, p. 2.

The survey dealt not only with spirituality as a general concept, but also with religious beliefs and affiliations and with attitudes toward life after this life. This report will summarize just a few of the key findings that are relevant to hospice care.

One opinion expressed in the survey results is that, due to the advancement of medical technology, the process of dying has become more depersonalized and is often treated as only a biomedical event. However, those who are dying are more than objects of medical attention; they remain human beings with the same wide variety of needs as those experienced over the course of their life—emotional, spiritual, as well as medical (Gallup, 1997, p. 3).

A portion of the national survey focused on how the respondents might derive comfort in their dying days. The main attitude they expressed is the need for companionship and spiritual support. A majority identified comfort in the form of human contact; it would be important to them to have someone with whom they can share fears or concerns. Forty-seven percent identified having someone holding their hand or touching them as a means of providing comfort.

When asked about spiritual comfort, 44 percent said that it would be very important to have someone help them become spiritually at peace. However, the types of support related to spiritual care were quite varied, including praying alone, praying with someone, having someone pray for them, touching, allowing the patient space and privacy, and other types of support drawn from people with a wide variety of spiritual beliefs. This demonstrates how caregivers need to be aware that sensing the identification of spiritual needs will likely vary among hospice patients.

Although it is natural that people look to their family or friends during difficult times (such as the dying process), it was interesting to learn that far less than a majority of respondents said that they would likely turn to a member of the clergy for comfort. Eighty-one percent said they would more likely look to family and 61 percent to friends for comfort during their dying days. Only 36 percent said that a member of the clergy would be comforting in many ways, which is close to the percentage (30 percent) who felt that way toward a doctor or nurse.

The survey respondents expected medical competency from their physician, but a strong majority (68 percent) said that it is important to have a doctor who cares about them, and they were almost equally clear (54 percent) on wanting a doctor who knows them well. This is significant to hospice caregivers due to the amount of time that is usually spent with each patient, and it supports the theories on the importance of spiritual care expressed by Kearney (1990) and Sheehan (1997).

Another interesting finding of the survey showed evidence that persons with little interest in spiritual matters would choose to relieve pain at the cost of shortening life.

CONCLUSIONS

As a volunteer for the Milwaukee Hospice Residence, I have experienced that it can be difficult to take care of people during the dying process. Accurately assessing patient needs and meeting those needs can sometimes be next to impossible. Providing spiritual care has its own very unique challenges.

One important consideration is that the definition of spirituality is very likely different in some way for each person. Labeling someone as having less interest in spirituality could deny that person the kind of care that may not be religious in nature, but that nevertheless might address the fundamentals of the human spirit.

After researching this topic, I found some comfort in learning that almost everyone is capable of providing spiritual care, even if their religious background is limited. In some cases, a limited background in religion actually can be advantageous, because providing spiritual care may not rely solely on religious theories, commitment, or practices. However, that is not to underestimate the importance of becoming familiar with basic theories and practices associated with organized religions, primarily because their doctrines and practices may play an important part in a patient's life. In hospice care, patient care takes a wholistic approach, so it is inevitable that questions of religion and spirituality will surface.

When a patient does look to a caregiver for support, three important considerations must be kept in mind. First, and probably the most important, is that the caregiver must listen without bias or prejudgment. It is human nature to hold prejudices and want to impose personal beliefs and values on others. However, that is not an appropriate role for a hospice caregiver. With the vastly different individuals who enter hospice care, it is not realistic to think that each patient will share the same value system as each (or any) member of the hospice team.

Second, hospice caregivers should not feel a need to answer spiritual questions for patients. Instead, it is the role of the hospice team to create an environment that facilitates spiritual growth and healing. This can be achieved simply by holding a patient's hand or sitting quietly by his or her side, being available in case of the need for someone to listen.

Finally, it is important for hospice caregivers to be open to discussing and learning about issues related to spirituality and even religion. Hospice centers on the idea that the human being is made up of mind, body, and spirit. To treat one dimension without regard to the others is not consistent with wholistic care and the hospice philosophy. Becoming comfortable with providing spiritual care tells the hospice patient, as stated by Dame Saunders (1975), "You matter to the last moment of your life," a statement so eloquent that it has been used as a slogan for NHO literature.

REFERENCES

Carr, W. (1995). Spiritual care and healing in the hospice. *America* 174(4, August 12): 26-29.

Flood, C. (1984). Evolution of hospice. *The American Journal of Hospice Care* 1(1):1, 15-17.

George H. Gallup International Institute (1997). Spiritual beliefs and the dying process: Key findings from a national survey conducted for the Nathan Cummings Foundation and the Fetzer Institute. Princeton, NJ: GH Gallup International Institute.

Kearney, Michael (1990). Spiritual pain. *The Way: Contemporary Christian Spirituality* 30(1):47-54.

Munly, A. (1983). *The hospice alternative.* New York: Basic Books.

Nathan Cummings Foundation (1998). Detailed findings: Finding comfort in their dying days. *Spiritual beliefs and the dying process: A report on a national survey,* pp. 1-8 [online]. Available: <http://www.ncf.org/ncf/publications/reports/feltzer/detailedfindingsa.html>.

NHO (1996). *Hospice: A special kind of caring.* Arlington, VA: National Hospice Organization.

Saunders, C. (1975). *I was sick and you visited me.* London: St. Christopher's Hospice.

Sheehan, M. (1997). Spirituality and care at the end of life. *Choices: The newsletter of the choice in dying* 6(2):1-3. Available: <http://www.choices.org>.

Chapter 9

Integrating Spirituality in Counseling with Older Adults

Ann Driscoll-Lamberg

It is estimated that by the year 2030, almost 20 percent of the population will be over sixty-five years of age (*White House Paper,* 1995, p. 1). With such a large influx of people into the geriatric population and the limited resources available for serving it, mental health professionals need to explore all options open to older adults. One area that has been ignored in the past is spirituality.

RESEARCH FINDINGS

Recent gerontological research suggests that the majority of the current cohort of older adults value religion and are active in their religious practice. A 1994 Gallup poll conducted by the Princeton Religion Research Center found that 76 percent of persons over age sixty-five regarded religion as highly important in their lives. Fifty-two percent reported attending religious services on a weekly basis (Baker and Nussbaum, 1997).

In a study of 106 persons at a typical geriatric assessment center, 90.5 percent stated they believed in a personal God and 71.5 percent reported praying once a day or more. It was reported that 71.5 percent had two or more of their closest five friends as members of their congregation and 54.4 percent attended worship once a week or more (Baker and Nussbaum, 1997). It is evident that religion plays a large role in the lives of older adults.

Significant losses come with aging, whether they are actual or perceived. These include diminished social resources, such as friends and family who die or move away. Retirement brings a loss of role and identity, and there can be significant physical decline and illness that affect an older adult's ability to function independently. The older adult may have feelings of low self-esteem, loss of love, and lost value to others. These significant losses often lead to depression or anxiety. The one compensating resource everyone has access to is religion. Historically, it has been the human response to the problem of helplessness and loss of control in almost every culture (Gerson, 1998).

At the 1995 White House Conference on Aging, it was stated that of the 32 million Americans age sixty-five and over, nearly five million suffer from persistent symptoms of depression, and over one million have major depression (*White House Paper,* 1995). With such a high percentage of depressed elders, health care providers need to come up with coping mechanisms and methods of treating and assisting these individuals with coping mechanisms. One way to do this is to include spirituality as a part of treatment.

Significant research has been conducted on the relationships between mental health and religion (see Chapter 4), as well as on the generally positive effects religion has on coping. Several scholars have found that, compared to nonreligious elders, older persons who are religious have better functional health and higher levels of adjustment as indicated by lower levels of mortality, depression, suicide, anxiety, and alcohol abuse. Koenig (1997) reported that his research group conducted a study in the late 1980s sponsored by the National Institute on Aging. They surveyed 4,000 persons in central North Carolina to determine whether those who are more religiously active would be more or less depressed than those who were not religious. The results showed that those who attended church at least once a week were only about half as likely to be depressed as those who attended church less frequently. The results held regardless of age, sex, race, level of social support, or degree of physical illness or functional disability (Koenig, 1997, pp. 58-59).

Morse and Wisocki (1987) examined the extent to which religious beliefs and church attendance influence psychological adjustment in later life. The study was done with 156 persons over age sixty who were recruited from western Massachusetts senior centers. The participants were asked questions related to their religiosity and then given the Mood Adjective Checklist. Those with high religiosity scores were significantly less likely to be depressed and anxious; they also reported less psychosomatic illness, phobia, and aggression than did subjects with low religiosity scores. The study concluded that elderly people with higher levels of religious activity and beliefs show better psychological health and adjustment (Morse and Wisocki, 1987).

Pargament and colleagues (1990) asked 586 church members from ten mainstream Protestant and Catholic congregations to describe a negative event that happened during the previous year and to indicate how they coped with it through religious and nonreligious coping activities. They found that religious coping variables were significant predictors of positive outcomes. Religious coping activities predicted outcomes more strongly than traditional dispositional religious variables and nonreligious coping variables. The coping variables included those that stress an individual's personal and living relationship with God. Spiritually based activities or those focusing on a personal relationship with God related the most strongly to positive outcomes. Belief in a loving and just God, the experience of God as supportive, involvement in religious rituals, and a search for spiritual and personal support through religion were all associated with positive outcomes. Coping with problems through religious faith and activities appears to buffer individuals from the negative impact of medical problems more effectively than even the typical forms of counseling (Baker and Nussbaum, 1997).

Nelson (1990) examined the association between religious orientation, depression, and self-esteem among sixty-eight elderly participants of a day care program in Austin, Texas. The Geriatric Depression Scale measured depression, the Rosenberg Self-Esteem Scale measured self-esteem, and religious orientation was measured by a modified version of the Allport and Ross Religious Orientation Scale, developed in 1967. There was a significant inverse correlation between intrinsic religiosity and both depression and low self-esteem (those who were highly religious had fewer instances of depression and of low self-esteem). Also, a nonsignificant but positive trend related low church attendance to both depression and low self-esteem (Nelson, 1990).

A study of 131 elderly residents in a southern Florida apartment facility was done by Johnson and Mullins (1989). They compared the effects of involvement in various types of family and friendship relationships on loneliness, a psychological construct related to depression and unhappiness. After controlling for other factors, they found that a greater involvement in the social aspects of religion was significantly more likely to be related to the absence of loneliness than was social involvement in either family or friendships (Johnson and Mullins, 1989).

ASSESSING SPIRITUALITY

It is evident that counselors, social workers, and other mental health professionals should be assessing older adults' spiritual needs and possibly using spiritual tools during counseling sessions. In the past, most mental health professionals did not receive training in regard to spirituality. References to spirituality and religion were not discussed or taught in relation to practice. This has been an obstacle for many professionals, but spirituality is starting to play a role in the mental health field.

Another obstacle among many clinicians has been their discomfort in discussing religion or spirituality. Clinicians must become comfortable with the topic. This can be difficult because their professional training may have fostered the idea that the topic was not valuable or should be avoided (Bracki et al., 1990).

The importance of religion for older adults has been well established, so it is critical for mental health professionals to begin the process of utilizing each person's belief system, faith, or spirituality for understanding the person and providing subsequent treatment (Bracki et al., 1990).

It is important to note that some people claim to be spiritual without a focus on God and the beliefs and activities frequently associated with religion.

> These individuals are able to feel a sense of spiritual connectedness within themselves through memory and imagination; they also experience integrative powers of spirituality in their relationships with others and the world. (Baker and Nussbaum, 1997, p. 38)

Many older adults experience a strong connection between their religious faith and a sense of spirituality (Baker and Nussbaum, 1997).

When mental health professionals work with older adults, they need to become aware of their clients' spiritual needs. Yet only rarely is a thorough spiritual assessment done. This author reviewed various assessment tools used by mental health professionals in Milwaukee, Wisconsin, including the Community Options Program Assessment, the Nursing Home Minimum Data Set, and two assessment tools used by geriatric clinics. All of the assessment tools asked clients what religion they were practicing, but none asked any questions relating to their spiritual needs.

By ignoring the spiritual component, mental health professionals fail to focus on the whole person, missing much strength for coping with adversity and loss, as well as a support system important enough to help enhance the quality of life (Bracki et al., 1990). Therefore a spiritual assessment should be made alongside the psychosocial assessment when interviewing clients.

Bergin and Richards (1997) give five reasons a religious-spiritual assessment should be done when working with clients. It can

1. help therapists better understand their clients' worldviews and therefore increase the capacity to empathetically understand and work with them;
2. determine if the client's religious-spiritual orientation is healthy or unhealthy and what impact that may have on the individual's presenting problems and disturbance;
3. determine whether a client's religious-spiritual beliefs and community could be used as a resource to help them better cope, heal, and grow;
4. determine which spiritual interventions could be used in therapy to help their clients; and
5. determine whether clients have unresolved doubts, concerns, or needs that should be addressed in therapy. (pp. 172-174)

As reported by Ellor (1999), Douglas Olson gives eight common variables that should be included in a religious-spiritual assessment. The clients should be asked for their

1. relationship to a church or spiritual community (e.g., What is their spiritual support?);
2. religious history, organizational practice, and degree of commitment to religion/spirituality;

3. degree of formal participation within an organized setting;
4. degree of commitment to their belief system;
5. private daily spiritual experiences of the client outside of organized religion;
6. values and ethical precepts that give a sense of responsibility and respect for human dignity expressed as a product of spiritual life;
7. spiritual and religious beliefs and their development to date; and
8. comfort and strength gained from religion or spirituality.

APPLYING SPIRITUALITY TO PRACTICE

Once mental health professionals have assessed a client's spiritual needs, there are many ways to meet those needs in one's practice. First, a spiritual assessment is a tool for the practitioner to get a complete understanding of the client's spiritual needs. Then the clinician can use the assessment to refer the client for the appropriate service, such as pastoral care or a parish nurse. Simply finding him or her a ride to church or other religious services can help a client.

A spiritual assessment may help the practitioner understand why a client is reacting or behaving a certain way. For example, a social worker had a ninety-two-year-old woman with dementia who refused to participate in card games and bingo at a day care center. It was only when the social worker found out that the client was a Southern Baptist who believed it was not appropriate to play gambling games that the reason for her refusal was explained. The practitioner then was able to teach the day care staff how to work with the woman.

Activities such as sacred readings and praying with clients may help them find comfort and hope in their therapeutic process. Hospice patients may find comfort in Scripture and prayer as they face their own mortality. Scripture or sacred readings have been used frequently by psychotherapists. The therapist may quote Scripture to clients, interpret Scripture to them, relate stories from Scripture that pertain to a client's situation, or encourage their own Scripture reading (Bergin and Richards, 1997, p. 209). Research shows that some therapists use prayer in sessions, whether praying for a client or praying with a client (Bergin and Richards, 1997, p. 203).

Meditation, guided imagery, and centering activities allow individuals to get in touch with their personal feelings and focus on their problems. Centering is a reflective process that gives the participant access to his or her unique human spirit.

Life review or reminiscence, which is a cognitive process of recalling events from the past that are personally significant and perceived as reality based, is helpful for clients who feel depressed or have feelings of worthlessness (Kovach, 1991). Reminiscence is a source of self-referent knowledge. It directly influences a person's sense of self-worth by contributing to the construction and reconstruction of knowledge about the self. Self-esteem directly influences feelings of satisfaction with life while reinforcing adaptive behaviors (Kovach, 1991).

Journaling can assist a client in sorting out feelings and letting out emotion by writing down one's feelings. Discussing values and morals that stem from religious beliefs may also play a role in therapy. For example, forgiving is an act that has important spiritual consequences. In the Christian tradition, forgiveness is believed to restore people's relationship with God, help them receive the gift of salvation, demonstrate their faith in God and in Jesus Christ, and show their desire to do God's will (Bergin and Richards, 1997, p. 212).

CONCLUSION

Research shows that religion and spirituality are important to older adults and that religion and spirituality have predominantly positive effects on an individual's mental health and coping abilities. Therefore it is imperative that a spiritual assessment be done when working with geriatric clients. Because it is an integral part of themselves and their lives, practitioners should provide spiritual counseling in their own practices or refer their clients to appropriate professional persons or spiritual care services.

REFERENCES

Baker, D. and Nussbaum, P. (1997). Religious practice and spirituality—Then and now: A retrospective study of spiritual dimensions of residents residing at a continuing care retirement community. *Journal of Religious Gerontology* 10(3):33-44.

Bergin, A. and Richards, P.S. (1997). *A Spiritual strategy for counseling and psychotherapy.* Washington, DC: American Psychological Association.

Bracki, M., Thibault, J., Netting, E., and Ellor, J. (1990). Principles of integrating spiritual assessment into counseling with older adults. *Generations* 14(4)55-58.

Ellor, J. W. (1999). *Spiritual assessment: A survey of constructive elements and issues.* March 25 Lecture Handout, Marquette University.

Gerson, D. (1998). Successful aging: Focus on public policy and spiritual well-being. *Journal of Religious Gerontology* 10(4):64-75.

Johnson, D. P. and Mullins, L. C. (1989). Religiosity and loneliness among the elderly. *Journal of Applied Gerontology* 8(1):110-131.

Koenig, H. (1997). *Is religion good for your health? The effects of religion on physical and mental health.* Binghamton, NY: The Haworth Press.

Kovach, C. (1991). Reminiscence: Exploring the origins, processes, and consequences. *Nursing Forum* 26(3):14-19.

Morse, C. K. and Wisocki, P. A. (1987). Importance of religiosity to elderly adjustment. *Journal of Religion and Aging* 4(1):15-27.

Nelson, P. B. (1990). Intrinsic/extrinsic religious orientation of the elderly: Relationship to depression and self-esteem. *Journal of Gerontological Nursing* 16(2):29-35.

Pargament, K. I., Ensing, D. S., Falgout, K., Olsen, H., Reilly, B., Van Haitsma, K., and Warren, R. (1990). God help me: Religious coping efforts as predictors of the outcomes of significant negative life events. *American Journal of Community Psychology* 18:793-824.

White House Paper on Mental Health, Substance Abuse, and Aging. (1995). Washington, DC: White House Conference on Aging. Available on the Internet at <www.pub. whitehouse.gov>.

Chapter 10

Spirituality in Social Work Practice with Older Persons

Derrel R. Watkins

The term spirituality, when used in conjunction with social services, is often viewed as a contradiction by many professional social workers. In a survey of spiritual care delivered by hospice teams, Babler (1995, pp. 58-59) found that social workers were the least likely to self-report that they provided such care. Some social work professionals seem to think that anything spiritual belongs exclusively to the religious sector of the community and therefore is not the purview of professional social workers. Others, in more recent years, have attempted to broaden the term to include attitudes, emotions, and behaviors that are religious. Many have the erroneous notion that social work and spirituality have never been related to each other.

A quick review of the history of social work, nevertheless, reveals that social work was founded in the context of the spiritual-religious domains of societies in Europe and America. The streams of history that fed into the founding of modern social work as a profession include, almost exclusively, religious organizations. Casework, for example, grew out of two religiously based social service delivery systems: The charity organization societies of England and America were begun by a minister in Glasgow, Scotland, and brought to America by an Episcopal minister (Fink, Anderson, and Conover, 1968, pp. 34-39; Lewis, 1971). Another was the Daughters of Charity begun by Father Vincent DePaul in France (Watkins, 1994, p. 17).

Contemporary social group work and community organization draw upon the settlement house movement begun by churchmen in England

and brought to America by church-related groups. Almost all of these continued to offer spiritual-religious services as a part of their social services programming. Hull House in Chicago, for example, offered religious services as part of its social service package from its very beginning in 1889 (Davis, 1977).

The value premise upon which social work is practiced has significant spiritual overtones. The conviction of the inherent worth, integrity, and dignity of persons; the belief in the right to self-determination; the belief in equal opportunity for all, limited only by the individual's capabilities; and social responsibility of persons, all speak to the spirituality of persons (Friedlander, 1976, pp. 1-6). This value premise is seen by many as parallel to what is known as the Judeo-Christian Ethic.

DEFINITION OF SPIRITUAL AND SPIRITUALITY

The term spiritual, as I use it here, includes the inner resources and ultimate concern of older persons. It provides the basic value around which all other values are evaluated; the persons' central philosophy of life—religious, nonreligious, or antireligious—that provides direction for their attitudes and behaviors. It includes the quality of life in which there is a cohesiveness, integrity, and wholeness that goes beyond the basic level of physical and psychosocial needs and relationships. It may include issues related to supernatural and nonmaterial dimensions of what it means to be human (Moberg, 1984; Babler, 1995, p. 40). Social workers have long recognized that people expend a significant amount of psychological and physical energy engaging these issues, but a significant number have not recognized them as pertaining to spirituality.

Social work educators Ellor, Netting, and Thibault (1999, pp. 6-7) define the term spirituality as an individual's unique spiritual "style." They explain that it refers to the way persons seek, find, create, use, and expand personal meaning in the context of their universe. This conceptual statement should be useful in that it can enable social workers to more precisely determine what is spiritual care in distinction from what is simply psychological or emotional. Indeed, a side benefit to psychological care may be that persons experience a form of spiritual care as well. It is very likely that the reverse is also true.

One of the problems researchers experience is the blurring of lines between what is spiritual and what is psychological. This should not be surprising in that the word psychology is drawn from an ancient word that literally means the study of the soul or spirit. It is therefore understandable that some significant overlap would occur between the concern for people's "psyche" and their spirituality.

I cannot recall a time in my study and practice of social work that we did not emphasize holistic approaches to assessment and treatment in the delivery of social services with any population. This usually means that assessment and treatment planning must include cognition, emotion, and volition. People's circumstances should be evaluated in light of their own abilities, their family contexts, and their social environments. The academic disciplines that inform social workers, enabling these assessments, are psychology, sociology, social psychology, biology, economics, and political science. Although all of these disciplines are important, we are missing one of the most important elements in assessment if we avoid the spiritual.

The spiritual dimension of people's lives affects each of the domains of living: physical, mental-emotional, relational, economic, and communal. Each of these, in turn, has an impact upon the spiritual. Jane Thibault (1993, pp. 1-20), a social worker and clinical gerontologist with the School of Medicine at the University of Louisville, for example, discusses a case of an older woman whose symptoms pointed to clinical depression. Her assessment, however, revealed that the woman was bored with her church and other aspects of her relationship with her God. As a result her life had lost its meaning and purpose. When she was able to renew her relationship with her God in the context of her religious experience, her depression went into remission. This illustrates one of the important contributions that recognizing the value of spirituality can have for the social worker and the client system.

THE IMPORTANCE OF SPIRITUAL CARE
BY SOCIAL WORKERS

Religion and spirituality are important parts of the everyday lives of older persons. If this fact is lost to social workers, they miss an opportunity to link older clients to a major source of strength for coping and for support systems that serve to enhance the quality of their lives (Bracki et al., 1990). Psychiatrist Harold Koenig (1994, pp. 283-295) of the Duke University School of Medicine suggests that mental health professionals would benefit from recognizing that both healthy and physically ill older persons experience a wide range of spiritual needs. Space does not allow for an in-depth discussion, but the list includes a need for meaning, purpose, and hope; a need to transcend circumstances; a need for support in dealing with loss; a need for continuity; a need for validation and support of religious behavior; a need to engage in religious behaviors, a need for personal dignity and sense of worthiness; a need for unconditional love; a need to express anger and doubt; a need to feel that God is on their side; a need to love and serve others; a need to be thankful; a need to forgive and be forgiven; and a need to prepare for death and dying.

Older persons often expect any professional who has concern for their personal well-being to understand their spiritual along with physical, economic, and social needs. Greene (1986) underscores one aspect of this issue when she says, "The need for social affiliation, place, and recognition is very powerful and persists throughout the life cycle" (p. 119). Social workers who understand the value of spirituality for persons, especially older ones, can be very helpful to them.

Although, in most rural and small town communities, a majority of older persons turn to their ministers for help more often than to any other professional, there are significant groups of older persons who may not have the access or desire to talk with a spiritual care professional. They will, however, want and need to talk with someone who understands. Urban dwellers may turn to their ministers less frequently, but their spiritual needs are often even more acute.

Acknowledging the full continuum of care requires that social workers recognize those attributes that have always given older persons a sense of meaning and purpose in life. That which has been experienced as meaningful earlier in life should be recognized as a source of strength and support in the later years. This understanding becomes even more acute when the mental health professional is attempting to determine whether or not the client system is using religion in a healthy or psychopathological manner (Bracki et al., 1990).

When clients encounter circumstances or find themselves in environments that are strange or life threatening, they experience a great deal of anxiety. For most, this leads to questions that are basically spiritual in nature. In settings such as hospitals, nursing homes, retirement communities, and community-based senior citizen centers, social workers and nurses are the professionals most likely to be confronted with a patient/client's spiritual needs (Shelly and Fish, 1988, pp. 157-182).

Social workers often speak of wholistic practice but regularly segment client systems. For example, they refer physically ill persons to physicians or nurse practitioners, persons with legal problems to lawyers, and persons with spiritual needs to ministers or chaplains. It is appropriate to do so in many, if not most, cases. This, however, does not preclude social workers from discussing spiritual needs with older clients. Social workers are often expected to discuss medical and legal needs with their clients, and they should not hesitate to discuss spiritual needs at the same level of concern. Referral is appropriate when the needs discussed require a level of expertise that is beyond the worker.

There are, however, many social workers whose training prepared them to specialize in medical social work, and others in public policy. A smaller number are trained in church or religiously based practice. A number of graduate schools of social work have arrangements with schools of theology, whereby students may earn a degree in theology and a degree in social work at the same time. A larger number of undergraduate programs are located in religiously funded colleges and universities where they may include theological courses in their degree programs. It is not necessary, however, for social workers to have specific specializations in any of these fields to practice in settings where they may be confronted with these various needs. This is one reason why wholistic training has been promoted by social work educators and professional organizations. To be truly wholistic the social worker must have an understanding of all of the domains of living. This includes the spiritual along with the physical and mental. It is important that social workers not address only part of the client's needs and ignore or avoid such an important aspect of her or his life.

HOW SPIRITUAL CARE IS DELIVERED
BY SOCIAL WORKERS

Social workers have historically practiced their profession under the auspices of an agency that delivers human services to specified segments of the general public. Some agencies deliver comprehensive services to a wide spectrum of persons with a variety of problems. Some target a specific part of the population and deliver a much more specialized group of social services, such as child welfare, youth services, and services to senior citizens. In recent decades many social workers, following the model of medicine and law, have set up private-practice offices. Many in private practice specialize in family therapy or family intervention. Some deliver counseling services to older individuals and families. Those who practice under the auspices of an agency that draws its financial support from tax monies or from cooperative charity funding such as United Way, may have restrictions on whether or under what conditions they provide spiritual care. The legal parameters of licensing agencies, and their own ethical codes, restrict those who are in private practice.

In general, social workers approach intervention with older persons from three perspectives: primary, secondary and tertiary (Beaver and Miller, 1992, pp. 32-119). *Primary social work* suggests that where a possibility of some type of dysfunction exists, social work interventions attempt to prevent them or to minimize their effect. *Secondary social work* engages in treating persons with dysfunctional conditions. *Tertiary social work* assesses the need for services that are limited or not available to older persons and organizes groups and communities to provide them. In addition, social workers assess the roles of agencies, policies, rules, and regulations that may be causing problems for some older persons, and they are advocates for social change.

In *primary interventions,* spiritual care is provided by social workers when they recognize that a condition exists in which essential spiritual resources are either diminishing for clients or are functionally absent. The worker then attempts to restore those resources or finds adequate replacements. For example, Mrs. Jones, who is eighty-seven, looks forward to attending her senior adult Sunday school class at the Baptist church each Sunday morning. Recently she has been unable to attend because she can no longer drive her own car. Her spiritual well-being is enhanced by her relationship with her friends in the class and she draws spiritual strength and renewal from the study of the Bible along with the worship services. The social worker at the retirement home where she lives has heard about her difficulty and arranged for the home's van to transport her to and from her class meetings and worship services. This was essentially a "needs-providing" intervention and, at least for the time being, it was effective.*

In another case, Mr. Clinton's eyesight was failing so he could no longer read his newspaper and Bible. He remarked to the social worker that he had made it a practice to read his Bible every day and now he felt a loss because he could no longer continue doing what had been a significant source of spiritual refreshment to him. The social worker stopped by the public library and found that The Library of Congress makes audiotapes available, free of charge, to persons who are sight impaired. They provide both the audiotapes and the tape player. The social worker, with Mr. Clinton's permission, placed the order. Soon a set of audiotapes that contained the complete Bible along with a tape player were delivered to Mr. Clinton.

Secondary spiritual care requires a more intense involvement with the client system. It involves both problem-solving and conflict-resolving interventions. Problem-solving interventions suggest that social workers enable client systems to recognize the nature and scope of the problem, sort through possible solutions, and make decisions regarding the most viable alternatives leading to a solution. For example, Robert Mitchell, a social worker at the county general hospital, met with Mrs. Lewis and her son and daughter to work out a solution to Mrs. Lewis' living arrangements so that she could be released from the hospital. She did not want to go to a nursing home. Her son and daughter each had a room at home that could be used for their mother, but they were employed in low-wage jobs and could not afford to hire a day nurse for her care while they were working. As with many family caregivers, they earned too much money to qualify for public assistance, but not enough to pay their rent, utilities, food, and clothing bills while also hiring help for persons dependent on them.

---

*The names of Mrs. Jones and other examples described in this chapter are fictional. They are composites of a number of cases I have known. None identifies any specific person.

Their primary problem with placing Mrs. Lewis in a nursing home was a spiritual one. Their church taught that it was the spiritual duty of the children to care for their aging parents. Mrs. Lewis expected them to do so, as well. In the interview Mr. Mitchell discovered that Mrs. Lewis had been active as a member of the church's evangelistic team until her illness and that she valued her ability to witness about her faith. Mr. Mitchell had a basic understanding of her religion and suggested that she might have a choice: She could stay at her son's home with the help of a companion service worker. In such an arrangement she would not see very many people with whom she could share her faith. On the other hand, she could move to an extended-care facility where she would be in contact with many people where her witness would be extended. In a real sense she would continue to be involved in what she felt was her most important service to her God. The whole family supported her decision to move to the extended-care facility.

Conflict resolution often calls for very sophisticated intervention on the part of the social worker. There are times when an apparent psychiatric problem is, in fact, a spiritually based problem that is affecting an older person's mental health. For example, Mrs. Friedman came to the Jewish senior citizen center to talk with the social worker, Mrs. Levine, about her problem of living alone in her home. She no longer felt like eating and taking baths, and the television programs were getting boring. She had quit attending Sabbath services at her synagogue. She was angry with God for taking all her family away in death and leaving her to live alone with her memories. She was withdrawing from almost all social contact although she knew that this was not in her best interest.

Mrs. Levine began to ask questions that would help determine if Mrs. Friedman was experiencing a form of clinical depression. They discussed the possibility of a referral to a psychiatrist or the local hospital's mental health clinic, or, as a temporary alternative, involvement with a Jewish older women's group, led by Mrs. Levine, that was dealing with ways of managing depression. Mrs. Friedman indicated that she was not sure she wanted to tell these other women about her "problems with God." She was not sure they would understand. She chose the group, however, and soon found that all of the other women were expressing many of the same feelings. Her problem was not a clinical depression, but a functional depression that was fostered by her guilt about her hostile feelings toward God. Restoring her relationship with her God by working with a group from her own faith community was an effective intervention. (It is important to note that Mrs. Levine carefully monitored all of the persons in her care and made sure that each understood that the group was not a substitute for clinical treatment if or when it was needed.)

Tertiary intervention calls for social workers to examine the rules, regulations, and practices of government and private agencies. They need to determine if community agencies are adequately meeting the needs of older persons or if there are gaps in services that might cause social systems to fail. This includes the spiritual care systems along with others.

Although religious institutions in American society are expected to be the primary providers of spiritual care, they are not the only ones to whom older persons may turn when they have spiritual needs. In fact, according to recent surveys, a majority of Americans are not actively involved with any formal religious organization. This indicates that if their spiritual needs are not met through alternative sources, their spiritual well-being is at risk. For example, a number of persons who have their names on the membership roles of religious institutions rarely attend any regular programming. The only contact they have with a spiritual community may be at the senior center operated by the parks and recreation department of the city. Those who attend are the persons with whom they share meaning and purpose and who provide them with a sense of value and worth.

Some communities of older persons, such as those in inner-city neighborhoods, find that their religious institutions are no longer accessible to them. For some, the physical environment of the meeting place is a barrier. Restricted accessibility to the worship center and restrooms, dim or subdued lighting, uncomfortable temperature, height of seats, poor sound systems, slippery floors, timing of services, etc., can hinder the participation of many older persons. Still others may live in extended health care facilities, or are shut-ins unable to leave their homes to attend worship services.

Other problems may intrude. Take the case of Mrs. Norman, for example. She had been an active participant in her church for sixty-eight years. The church decided to move to a suburban location. Mrs. Norman and several other older women had counted on walking to worship services at their church when they could no longer drive. Now, there was no church of their denomination nearby. Mrs. Norman tried to attend a church of another denomination but the worship style was very foreign to her, and it did not meet her particular spiritual needs. A social worker at the local community recreation center heard the women talking. Although he was not of the same faith group, he called the priest of the church that had moved and convinced him to meet with the women and work out a plan whereby those who were left behind could be included in the ministry of the church.

In another case, a large retirement village did not provide for the worship needs of all of its residents. They encouraged local churches to use the meeting hall for worship, but the participation by local ministers was limited. Some of the residents were fortunate in that their churches provided transportation for any who wished to attend worship. Many residents, however, felt a strong need to participate in worship but were unable to do so because of the great distance to a church of their denomination. They were very disturbed that they could not observe the Eucharist each week. The social service director was alerted to the need when she attended a workshop at which a chaplain explained how important such observances were to many Christians. She immediately began to meet with Catholic and Anglican priests to work out a way to meet this need. She also met with the retirement center's administrative officers and submitted a proposal for the employment of a chaplain.

CAUTIONS TO OBSERVE
WHEN SPIRITUAL CARE IS DELIVERED
BY SOCIAL WORKERS

Three common pitfalls may confront social workers as they engage in the delivery of spiritual care to older client systems:

1. The temptation to persuade the older adult to accept the worker's religious understanding or theological persuasion
2. The tendency to avoid talking about spiritual and/or religious issues for fear of imposing the worker's own beliefs upon the older client
3. The possibility of replacing the older person's minister or priest as the primary spiritual advisor

Babler (1995, p. 40) suggests that spiritual care delivery involves allowing the view of spirituality held by the client system to be the framework for the intervention strategy used by the worker. One of the basic value premises for social work practice is that the client has the right to determine what her or his needs are and how they are to be met (Friedlander, 1976, pp. 1-6). To impose one's own religious or spiritual beliefs on a client would be a violation of professional ethics and poor social work practice.

From another perspective, to avoid dealing with religious or spiritual issues would seem to be poor practice as well. The worker, practicing basic social work skills, can be informed about the client's religious belief system by the client and then use that knowledge to assist the client system without violating the client's integrity. When social workers, or other professionals, avoid listening to clients talk about their religious beliefs, they may convey messages that say that the things clients want to deal with are not important. Clients may feel that the workers are imposing an agenda upon them that avoids one of the most important aspects of their lives. Research surveys reveal that religious and spiritual issues are considered very important to the daily lives of a majority of persons in America (Naisbitt and Aburdene, 1990, p. 275). Professionals who refuse to address these issues are considered by some to be either out of touch with reality or engaging in an arrogant form of practice (Moody, 1994).

Ethical values prohibit social workers from practicing medicine or law, if they do not have the proper professional credentials for practice in those fields. In the same manner, social workers who do not have the appropriate training and credentials in the ministry or priesthood would be wise not to usurp those roles when dealing with client systems. This does not preclude discussing matters of spirituality or religion from the client's perspective and enabling older persons to find resolutions to their questions or problems.

Some social workers have earned medical or law degrees and are licensed to practice those professions along with the practice of social work. Some, in like manner, have earned theology degrees and have been ordained by their respective religious bodies to practice as clergy. The practice setting (institution, agency, etc.) will usually define to what extent the social worker is expected to engage in a form of dual-professional practice. For example, some chaplains in retirement centers and nursing homes may have credentials in both professions and function in both roles.

While the practices of chaplaincy and social work have significant overlapping functions, agencies usually find it wise to clearly define the functional roles of each position. Social workers may find that they best serve the patient/client by providing basic spiritual care and referring the patient/client to a chaplain or the client/patient's own church ministers for specific spiritual guidance.

Another caution concerns cross-cultural practice with older persons from different nationalities and racial or ethnic identities. Persons with different cultural backgrounds may have subtle differences in the ways religious or spiritual practices are valued. Even if social workers read the literature about a particular religion or religious practice, they may not fully understand what the practice means to specific clients. Literature should be used primarily to help the worker to form pertinent questions that may aid client systems to communicate their concerns more precisely.

CONCLUSION

Spiritual care as a facet of social service delivery is of exceptional importance to the current aging cohort. Social work practice with older persons is enhanced when social workers become comfortable discussing spiritual and religious issues with their clients. Clients who benefit significantly from the practice of their religious beliefs receive more satisfying holistic services when workers enable them to find ways of accessing and growing in their spirituality. Even those clients who are not religious or who are opposed to religion, can benefit from spiritual care because it helps them deal with issues related to the meaning and purpose of their lives, connect with their inner resources, and find a sense of belonging or community.

Social workers, whether personally religious or not, can learn ways of helping clients to address spiritual issues in their lives, thus enhancing the effectiveness of social work practice. Assessment tools or instruments such as those included in the book by Ellor, Netting, and Thibault (1999), can guide social workers in dealing with client systems where questions of spirituality need to be addressed.

Maintaining an ethical professional practice is the primary guide for workers who are concerned with encroachment upon the older client's rights when the religious identification of the worker and client are different. At the heart of professional social work practice is a set of ethics that stresses the rights of clients to be protected from the imposition of the personal values and beliefs of the worker and/or agency. It would be unethical, for example, for a social worker, who is a Christian, to insist that a group that includes persons from Jewish, Muslim, and Hindu traditions participate in singing Christmas carols.

SUGGESTED READINGS

The following books and journals are resources a social worker might find especially useful when preparing to work with spiritual issues in the delivery of social services with older persons:

Bianchi, Eugene C. (1982). *Aging as a spiritual journey.* New York: Crossroad Publishing Company (reprinted in 1995).

Bullis, Ronald K. (1996). *Spirituality in social work practice.* Philadelphia: Taylor and Francis.

Canda, Edward R. (1998). *Spirituality in social work: New directions.* Binghamton, NY: The Haworth Press.

Canda, Edward R. and Leola Byrud Fuman. (1999). *Spiritual diversity in social work practice: The heart of helping.* New York: Free Press.

Ellor, James W. and Thomas R. Cole (Guest eds.) (1990). "Aging and the human spirit." *The Journal of the American Society on Aging* 14(4) (a special issue).

Ellor, James W., F. Ellen Netting, and Jane M. Thibault (1999). *Understanding Religious and spiritual aspects of human service practice.* Columbia, SC: The University of South Carolina Press.

Journal of Religious Gerontology, published quarterly by The Haworth Press.

Koenig, Harold G. (1994). *Aging and God: Spiritual pathways to mental health in midlife and later years.* Binghamton, NY: The Haworth Press.

Social Work and Christianity, published twice each year by the North American Association of Christians in Social Work.

Spirituality and Social Work (1999), published by the Council on
   Social Work Education.
Weaver, Andrew J., Harold G. Koenig, and Phyllis C. Roe (Eds.) (1998).
   Reflections on aging and spiritual growth. Nashville: Abingdon Press.

REFERENCES

Babler, John (1995). A comparison of spiritual care provided to hospice patients and
   families by hospice social workers, nurses, and spiritual care professionals. PhD dissertation. Fort Worth, TX: Southwestern Baptist Theological Seminary.
Beaver, Marion L. and Don A. Miller (1992). *Clinical social work practice with the elderly* (Second edition). Belmont, CA: Wadsworth Publishing Company.
Bracki, Marie A., Jane M. Thibault, F. Ellen Netting, and James W. Ellor (1990). Principles of integrating spiritual assessment into counseling with older adults. In *Generations: The Journal of the American Society on Aging* 14(4):55-58.
Davis, Allen F. (1977). Settlements: History. In *Encyclopedia of Social Work* (Seven-
   teenth issue, Volume 2) (pp. 1266-1271). Washington, DC: National Association of
   Social Workers.
Ellor, James W., F. Ellen Netting, and Jane M. Thibault (1999). *Understanding religious
   and spiritual aspects of human service practice.* Columbia, SC: University of South
   Carolina Press.
Fink, Arthur E., C. Wilson Anderson, and Merrill B. Conover (1968). *The field of social
   work* (Fifth edition). New York: Holt, Rinehart and Winston.
Friedlander, Walter A. (Ed.) (1976). *Concepts and methods of social work.* Englewood
   Cliffs, NJ: Prentice-Hall.
Greene, Roberta R. (1986). *Social work with the aged and their families.* New York:
   Aldine de Gruyter.
Koenig, Harold G. (1994). *Aging and God: Spiritual pathways to mental health in
   midlife and later years.* Binghamton, NY: The Haworth Press.
Lewis, Verl S. (1971). Charity organization society. In *Encyclopedia of Social Work*
   1(16):94-98. New York: National Association of Social Workers.
Moberg, David O. (1984). Subjective measures of spiritual well-being. In *Review of
   Religious Research* 25(4):351-364.
Moody, Harry R. (1994). Foreword: The Owl of Minerva. In Thomas, L. Eugene and
   Susan A. Eisenhandler (Eds.), *Aging and the religious dimension* (pp. ix-xv).
   Westport, CT: Auburn Press.
Naisbitt, John and Patricia Aburdene (1990). *Megatrends 2000.* New York: William
   Morrow and Company.
Shelly, Judith Allen and Sharon Fish (1988). *Spiritual care: The nurse's role* (Third
   edition). Downers Grove, IL: InterVarsity Press.
Thibault, Jane Marie (1993). *A deepening love affair: The gift of God in later life.* Nash-
   ville: Upper Room Books.
Watkins, Derrel R. (1994). *Christian social ministry.* Nashville: Broadman & Holman.

Chapter 11

Secular Franciscan Spirituality and Aging

Carol A. Nickasch

The purpose of this chapter is to investigate the relationship of "The Canticle of Brother Sun" by St. Francis of Assisi to the spiritual growth of the Secular Franciscans. It is based upon my experiences as one of its members for fifteen years and especially upon an introspective analysis of the role of spiritual development in the Secular Franciscan Order inspired by the poem "The Canticle of Brother Sun."

THE SECULAR FRANCISCAN ORDER

In the year 1221, the Third Order (now known as the Secular Franciscans) was officially established. In 1226, St. Francis sketched a rule of life for them in his letter to "All the Faithful" (Exhortation to the Brothers and Sisters of Penance). In the letter Francis spoke of the Gospel as being the source of salvation and life; anyone who put into practice the words of the Gospel would draw salvation from them.

Chapter 1 taught that as people of prayer and penance the Holy Spirit joins us to our Lord Jesus Christ. A person turned toward God follows the teaching and footsteps of our Lord Jesus Christ by responding to the inviting grace of God and living in union with Jesus with constant spiritual renewal, awareness of God's power and presence, and a promise of eternal happiness (Celano, 1972, p 37).

The Secular Franciscan Order remains active throughout the world. In the United States, as of spring 1999, there are 756 SFO Fraternities with 18,020 members, and 428,450 Secular Franciscan members in the world (TAU-USA, 1999). The spirituality of the Secular Franciscan is wrapped up in both the "Franciscan Spirit," which is Gospel to life and life to the Gospel, and the rituals that are performed by the secular. Some question how much is really spiritual and how much is more ritual. Those who follow Francis seem to be filled with peace, joy, and love.

The Secular Franciscan Order is alive today with a new Rule of Life approved by Pope Paul VI in 1978. This new rule captures the spirit of both the Second Vatican Council and the first rule of St. Francis. It consists of three chapters and states that every Secular Franciscan is "to observe the gospel of our Lord Jesus Christ by following the example of St. Francis of Assisi, who made Christ the inspiration and the center of his life with God and people" (Baldonado and Grant, 1981, pp. 49-50).

Secular Franciscans are as diverse in their fidelity to following Christ as their numbers are large. We are all committed to living in the world and to our family, job, and society. We are devoted as well to the Roman Catholic Church and to the special apostolates of our respective fraternities. The differences among the professed members of the Order reflect both the strength of our personal gifts and a genuine devotion to living the virtues of St. Francis in today's world. Whatever the pattern, however, we always look for and expect the gifts of peace, joy, and love. According to the new Rule of 1978, Chapter 1 describes the place of the Secular Franciscans within the Franciscan family and recognizes that laity, religious, and priests are all called to follow Christ in the footsteps of St. Francis.

Chapter 2 contains a thorough and detailed description of the Secular Franciscan way of life. Becoming a Secular Franciscan is an ongoing process that encourages the members to seek out others who embody the Spirit of Christ. It is the responsibility of each member to answer the call given to Francis to rebuild the Church. The members must continually seek out the sacrament of reconciliation as the privileged sign of the Father's mercy and the source of grace, while fully participating in the total sacramental life of the Church, above all the Eucharist. Secular Franciscans should develop a devotion to the Mother of Christ by imitating her life and example. They must detach themselves from excessive material wants and desires and lead a life of simplicity. The final section calls Secular Franciscans to develop a sense of community and fraternal life.

Chapter 3 describes the organization of the Secular Franciscan Order, which exists on four levels—local, regional, national, and international (Fonck, 1979).

FRANCISCAN SPIRITUALITY

Spirituality can be defined as a particular way in which to follow Christ. Differing spiritualities develop even within Catholicism because of the personality of each founder and their way of picturing who God is. Franciscan spirituality is simply to observe the Gospel. Franciscans strive to live the Gospel under seven rules according to the spirit of St. Francis that are a part of the initiation and formation of every Franciscan:

1. Being in communion with Christ, poor and crucified
2. Being in the love of the Father
3. Being in brotherhood with all people and all of creation
4. Participating in the life and mission of the church
5. Being continually in the process of conversion
6. Having a life of prayer, both private and public
7. Being an instrument of peace (Baldonado and Grant, 1981, p. 51)

Formation is an integral part of the spiritual growth and development of each Secular Franciscan. The process is well established. The part that may be lacking is the review of the writings of St. Francis and how those materials can be integrated into the daily life of a Secular Franciscan. Although all Franciscans read "The Canticle" (see Table 11.1), they do not necessarily internalize it and use it as a road map by which to live and prepare for death.

TABLE 11.1. The Canticle of Brother Sun

Most high, all-powerful, good Lord.

Yours are the praise, the glory and the honor and every blessing.

To you alone, Most High, they belong and no man is worthy

to pronounce your name.

Be praised, my Lord, with all your creatures,

especially Sir Brother Sun,

who is day and by him you shed light upon us.

He is beautiful and radiant with great splendor,

of you, Most High, he bears the likeness.

Be praised, my Lord, through Sister Moon and the Stars,

in the heavens you formed them clear and precious and beautiful.

Be praised, my Lord, through Brother Wind and through Air and Cloud and fair and all weather,

by which you nourish all that you have made.

Be praised, my Lord, through Sister Water,

who is very useful and humble and precious and pure.

Be praised, my Lord, through Brother Fire,

by whom you light up the night;

he is beautiful and merry and vigorous and strong.

Be praised, my Lord, through our Sister Mother Earth,

who sustains and guides us,

and produces diverse fruits with colored flowers and herbs.

Be praised, my Lord, by those who pardon for love of you,

and endure sickness and trials.

Blessed are they who shall endure them in peace,

for by you, Most High, they shall be crowned.

Be praised, my Lord, through our Sister Bodily Death,

from whom no man living can escape.

Woe to those who die in mortal sin.

Blessed are those, whom she will find in your most holy will,

Praise and bless my Lord and give him thanks and serve him with great humility.

St. Francis of Assisi, 1223 AD

FRANCISCAN SPIRITUAL GROWTH

Following the graduate seminar Spirituality and Aging, a question kept bothering me, "If a group had a prescription for spiritual growth and death, how would they view such a prescription?" Having been a professed Secular Franciscan for more than fifteen years, I believe that within the writings of St. Francis lies a prescription not only on how to live our daily lives, but also on how to accept pain, suffering, and death in the same spirit. I thought it was important to discover whether my fellow Franciscans felt the same way or if they had ever given any thought to that concept.

I designed a survey just to discover if there was a possibility that others may want to look at the writings of Francis and discover how to continue the process of spiritual growth. It consisted of four "yes" or "no" questions.

I then interviewed twenty-five Professed Secular Franciscans from two fraternities in the Milwaukee, Wisconsin, area. The ages ranged from thirty-five to the late eighties. Some had been Professed Franciscans only a short time, and others had been Professed for over fifty years. The results did not surprise me. The following are some of their responses.

Do you discover spiritual growth by studying the life of St. Francis?

- I always admired how St. Francis lived. I try to grow spiritually by following his example, but I do not always succeed.
- Yes. It was a turning point in my spiritual life when I became a fraternity member and began to follow in the footsteps of St. Francis.

Have you ever studied "The Canticle of Brother Sun" as a way to grow spiritually? If yes, did the study of the Canticle teach you how to live and prepare for death?

- Although I have not studied the Canticle, it does help one to grow in simplicity and to appreciate what God created for us.
- No, but I have access to spiritual books with prayers and a history of St. Francis.

- No. I've prayed it, but never really studied it.
- I have read it, not studied it, but it is a pure and simple way to live life and accept death.
- I haven't studied it, but I say it as a prayer often. It hasn't really phased me one way or the other.
- Yes. I read it but did not study it.

Do you think the Canticle written by St. Francis could be a guide to spiritual maturity and acceptance of death?

- Yes. Living by this will keep me in touch with God's grace.
- Yes. Sister Death becomes more real and less threatening.
- I have not studied this prayer. My growth spiritually as a Catholic, Christian, and a Franciscan prepares me not for death, but for resurrection.
- I tried to prepare for death and don't feel I'm afraid to die.
- Yes, it could be a guide, but it is not always easy to follow, especially in this world which is so materialistic and "me" orientated.
- Yes, I am glad it has been called to my attention. I'll be sure to look into it and read it regularly in my prayer life.
- Yes, very important for life going into the year 2000.
- Yes, probably if it were studied more. I am eighty years of age and returned to the Secular Franciscan order a year ago.

Never having studied the Canticle myself, I decided to investigate the reasons why Francis wrote the poem and what was happening in his own life. I felt this was important because if we truly follow in his footsteps, this would be an important aspect of his life and death. Could this poem become a guide for all Secular Franciscans to study, pray, and find peace in our own deaths? Conversion is a continuous process in the life of Francis and in those who follow his example. Because we are called to follow Francis, I believe that in the simplicity of the Canticle a person will discover the same spiritual growth, maturity, and guide to accept death as Francis did with perfect joy.

Written in the summer of 1223 during his last illness and amid intense suffering, the first part of the Canticle up to the verse about pardon was composed in the garden of the Poor Clares Convent at San Damiano where Francis also gave the poem a melody. The second part about pardon and peace was written after Francis was asked to restore peace to quarreling parties in a dispute between the civil and religious authorities of Assisi. The third part was written just before he died and displays a heart filled with joy and happiness. The deepest gratitude is toward Almighty God even for suffering and Sister Death (Celano, 1972, pp. 128-129).

One interminable night in the middle of winter, his pains became so terrible that he took pity on his poor Brother Body and prayed to God for the strength to bear the suffering. He found that his pain became the strong wind that bore his soul to God.

He said to a friar that for every trial on this earth, there is a joy in heaven; for every bitterness, a divine consolation; for every enemy who injures us, a creature who loves us. "This is a great grace and blessing given to us by God. Therefore, for His glory, for my consolation and the edification of my neighbor," he concluded, "I wish to compose a new song: 'Praises of the Lord, for his creatures.' These creatures minister to our needs every day. Without them, we could not live, yet through them the human race greatly offends the Creator. Every day we fail to appreciate so great a blessing by not praising, as we should the Creator and dispenser of all gifts" (Fortini, 1992, pp. 565-566). He was happy, with a sense of completion in having found the song that expressed the truth that he had been seeking from his earliest years (Fortini, 1992, p. 568).

The Canticle came at the climax of a long pilgrimage from his conversion and from total dependence on his Creator, which was marked by trials and struggles. The fact that the poem radiates light and serenity is proof that St. Francis has achieved a profound and complete reconciliation with the primal vital powers of his own psyche.

Spirituality in the Canticle

The Canticle could be regarded as the poetic expression of the reconciliation in man between the highest purpose (the quest of the most high) and the lower, obscure link with "mother earth," a poetic expression of the reconciliation between our "archeology" and our "teleology." St. Francis begins by addressing the Lord as "Most High." There can be no doubt but that this expresses a deep-rooted attitude of Francis's soul, his highest desire, and his thrust toward the divine. It is in Christ that Francis sees fully embodied the movement by which the soul renounces equality with the Most High and accepts its lowly roots in psyche, cosmos, and that fraternal presence to the world that becomes for it the pathway of spiritual ascent. For Francis, Christ is the true archetype, who "though he was in the form of God, did not deem equality with God something to be grasped at, rather he emptied himself and because of this, God highly exalted him" (Philippians: 2:6-11, New American Bible). The humiliation and exaltation of the most high Son of God was the central theme of Francis' meditations and around it he shaped his whole life. He summed up his religious ideals in these simple words, "to follow in the footsteps of your Son, our Lord, Jesus Christ, and so make our way to you, Most High, by your grace alone" (Leclerc, 1970, p. 34)

St. Francis declares blessed those who endure sickness and trials in peace, that is, in the calmness of order peace makes endurance a blessed thing because it places suffering in its true and only context, the creaturely existence of human beings. In our creaturehood we are beings-unto-death, and all suffering is a symbol of death. The most meaningful statement we can make about suffering is that it belongs to our existence as creatures. To endure it in peace is to understand the meaning of being a creature, to transform this understanding into wisdom by accepting and embracing our sufferings with love, and to rest serenely in the wisdom.

St. Francis greeted death with a loving salutation: "Welcome, my Sister Death," and in her company he made the last stage of his journey to Friar Christ. This simple and courageous attitude toward death is far removed from the ambiguity of our attitude to it (Doyle, 1981, p. 144). Throughout the centuries the followers of Christ have never forgotten that the heart of everything they are and do is their belief in the death and resurrection of Christ. In calling death his sister, Francis is reminding us that the Christian faith has a sacred message about human death (pp. 155-156). That faith is a way of interpreting the world, our own existence, and all reality.

SPIRITUAL INSPIRATION FROM ST. FRANCIS

As we continue on our journey, we realize our relationships with God, our neighbor and ourselves are of primary importance if we are to develop spiritually. As Francis looked on all of God's creatures, he felt an interconnectedness that became part of his daily life. Experiencing God in all things was his greatest desire. In the simplicity of prayer and meditation, we will find the same interconnectedness with all creatures.

Not only as Franciscans, but also as human beings, we too will experience trials and struggles. By placing our trust in the spirit of St. Francis, we will be able to look upon them as blessings and joys. Francis always praised God in everything he said and did. To win the greatest peace, we also must adopt the same attitude of praise and reconciliation. We need to spend time in our daily life centering ourselves in Christ. This comes by constantly emptying ourselves and allowing God and the Holy Spirit to work within us. (See Bodo, 1981 and Romb, 1969.)

Following his conversion, Francis emptied himself and wanted nothing more than to be with Christ. In Brother Sun, Francis saw the image of the loveliness of God as a symbol of constancy and permanence. The Sister Moon and the Stars were symbols of fluctuation and a series of changes that occur in our lives from conception to infancy, childhood to adolescence, and adulthood to old age. The Brother Wind is air in motion as invisible, though ever present and vital to our life; air is a powerful symbol of God, a symbol of God's grace.

Grace does not dispense with human nature, but perfects it. God will give each of us the grace we need to fulfill His plan for us on earth. Sister Water is useful, humble, precious, and pure integrity. Her presence demonstrates vividly that being has unity, truth, goodness, and beauty. Water also sanctifies. Brother Fire gives light and warmth to the world. Fire invokes a sense of awe. Sister Mother Earth gives the sense of belonging to it and of loving it deeply. Francis loved the earth because it was the fruit of God's free and loving decision to create it. Peace, pardon, and suffering are blessings that create a calmness of order.

The most meaningful statement we can make about suffering is that it belongs to our existence as creatures. To endure it in peace is to understand the meaning of a creature, to transform this understanding into wisdom by accepting suffering with love and to rest serenely in peace (Doyle, 1981, pp. 144-145).

CONCLUSION

In conclusion, I think there is a need to study in depth the role of the Canticle in the life of a Secular Franciscan. My conversations with those who completed the survey revealed that they were very anxious to learn more about the poem and wanted to know when I would come back and share my thoughts with them. As I reviewed the meanings of the symbols that Francis used, it became very clear that as Francis emptied himself, he was able to see all things as a response of God's love for us. The essence of who we are as Secular Franciscans is intertwined with the spirit of St. Francis.

As Secular Franciscans within the Roman Catholic Church, we are continually called to the conversion. The process of conversion means that we must always empty ourselves and be open to the Spirit of Christ in everything we do; this enables us to follow in the footsteps of St. Francis who followed in the footsteps of Christ. Formation within Secular Franciscan life is an ongoing process of studying the rule, the life of St. Francis, and the Gospel. As we are an aging group, we need to share with others the gift of our vocation. Because we are called to this vocation, we need to look seriously at how we can continue to grow within the Franciscan tradition. The ultimate challenge is to develop the attitude Francis had as he approached Sister Death, an attitude of acceptance and peace. Because many of our fraternity members are aging, they should study the Canticle. The Canticle could become a resource for them and others of how to view their own death. Will we be like Francis and embrace Sister Death?

REFERENCES

Baldonado, Felipe, O.F.M., and Zachary Grant, O.F.M. Cap. (1981). *The rule of the Secular Franciscan Order with a catechism and instruction.* Chicago: Franciscan Press.

Bodo, Murray, O.F.M. (1981). *The way of St. Francis: The challenge of Franciscan spirituality for everyone.* New York: Image Books.

Celano, Thomas (1972). *The first life of St. Francis: St. Francis of Assisi omnibus of sources.* Chicago: Franciscan Herald Press.

Doyle, Eric (1981). *St. Francis and the song of brotherhood.* New York: The Seabury Press.

Fonck, Benet A., O.F.M. (1979). *From gospel to life.* Chicago: Franciscan Herald Press.

Fortini, Arnaldo (1992). *Francis of Assisi.* New York: The Crossroad Publishing Company.

Leclerc, Eloi, O.F.M. (1970). *The Canticle of Creatures.* Chicago: Franciscan Herald Press.

New American Bible (1987). *St. Joseph Edition of the New American Bible.* New York: Catholic Book Publishing Co.

Romb, Anselm W., O.F.M. (1969). *Franciscan charism in the Church.* Patterson, NJ: St. Anthony Guild Press.

TAU-USA (1999). Budget report. National Fraternity, Secular Franciscan Order, (1999). Nuangola, PA: Secular Franciscan Publications.

Chapter 12

The Spiritual Life Review

David O. Moberg

Not very many generations ago, elders who seemed always to want to talk about their past were often considered to be a bit "off their rocker," experiencing "senility" or on the verge of a horrible mental condition that was inevitable if one lived long. Old age was viewed with bitter feelings of distaste, fear, and denial, as if it had little or no redeeming personal and social value. Today, influenced especially by the Pulitzer Prize-winning book *Why Survive? Being Old in America* by Butler (1975), the prominent psychiatrist who was the first director of the National Institute on Aging, the process of recounting and interpreting past life events is known to have mostly wholesome effects upon older persons and society (see Hendricks, 1999).

THE LIFE REVIEW

In a chapter on how old age had become "an absurdity, a time of life with virtually nothing to recommend it," Butler (1975, p. 402) summarized several characteristics and tendencies typical of older persons. One section presented the "Tendency Toward Life Review" (pp. 412-414), a concept he had coined by 1961. He reminded readers that reminiscence among older people is typically regarded as "a symptom, usually of organic dysfunction, and is felt to bespeak 'aimless wandering of mind' or 'living in the past' " (p. 413). Yet its value is evident in fascinating memoirs of great historical value composed during old age by gifted people and other examples in motion pictures and literature.

During a life review older people take stock of their own lives. "Life review provides a configuration, a mosaic of meaning in our lives, and facilitates the next stage which includes death. . . . [It] helps older adults tell their story, who they are and where they have been" (Kimble, 1995, p. 139). It reveals how the events, experiences, and circumstances of life fit into the frame of reference of a worldview and thus integrates them into a philosophy of life. The life review also makes many try to think and feel through what they will do with their remaining time and what material and emotional legacies they will give to others.

Autobiographical memoirs that summarize a person's life work and contributions can become treasured mementos among family members. They transmit family history and other knowledge and values to younger generations. Copies often become valuable additions to local, state, university, or organizational historical archives. Group discussions of such topics at senior center gatherings are interesting and therapeutic for all who attend.

Life-review therapy helps to reintegrate unresolved conflicts and fears, expiate guilt feelings, reconcile broken family relationships, and prepare the person for a peaceful death (Butler, 1975, pp. 412-413). Although used extensively by professional therapists, relatively untrained people who simply listen to others also help to meet social, emotional, and spiritual needs such as the psychological conflicts that have been reinforced by intermingled experiences of bereavement and grief, anger and sadness, anxieties and fears, and a sense of powerlessness from lack of control over many elements of one's fate.

The life review usually enhances the integrity of older adults, but it sometimes has the outcome of despair, an inability to accept one's fate and to face death realistically. Speculation about how different life would have been had other choices been made may flash into the minds of most elders, but some have extreme feelings of regret, frustration, discouragement, and meaninglessness that eliminate all thoughts of the accomplishments that also were present. "Reminiscence can be destructive to mental health if it involves brooding or obsessing on past negatives and prevents the elder from moving on. . . . [D]welling in the past can be used defensively to avoid taking responsibility and making needed changes in the here and now" (Koenig, 1994, p. 314n).

Some of the despair that occasionally accompanies one's life review emerges from unrealistic ideas about success in life. The cultural context that prizes youthfulness and demeans most features of aging contributes to feelings of lost self-worth. Unrealistic definitions of what they ought to have done with their lives bring disappointment to ordinary people. Comparisons with peers who boast of their actual or imagined achievements easily demean oneself. ("We do not dare to classify or compare ourselves with some who commend themselves. When they measure themselves by themselves and compare themselves with themselves, they are not wise," 2 Corinthians 10:12, NIV.)

Helping people see the optimistic side of their past and current circumstances and achievements can be a significant means of overcoming unbalanced pessimism. As Chaplain Ison (1998) has written, telling the story of one's life is like weaving a tapestry with symbolic ribbons of family, faith, health, hope, joy, death, love, adversity, and much more that creates "a weaving of great beauty, significance and holiness" (p. 3).

SPIRITUAL NEEDS IN LATE LIFE

Although every person is different, most people face a great deal of change during their later years. New joys and satisfactions come from opportunities for travel, time for hobbies, the lack of pressure to govern life by rigid schedules, grandchildren, and much more. At the same time, material, physical, social, and psychological needs are troublesome for many elders. Their health and strength are declining, relative income is diminishing under inflating prices of goods and services, friends are departing through death or moving to different communities, children and other family members are scattering, self-concepts may be changing, sometimes shattered through loss of roles by retirement from work or other meaningful positions, and they may feel the need to move to a safer, usually smaller, home.

Experiences such as those spill over into the spiritual domain that is so tightly interwoven with all the other areas of life, contributing to many spiritual needs. Shelly and Fish (1988) suggest that all spiritual needs fit under three main categories: meaning and purpose, love and relatedness, and forgiveness. Connected with them, however, are other practical, social, and psychological issues as people cope with the transitions, losses, anxieties, fears of dying and death, and blows to self-conceptions encountered in varying degrees by every aging person, all of which contribute to spiritual problems. The list of interconnected spiritual needs therefore can be extended to include the following overlapping categories.

The Need for Meaning and Purpose

The need for meaning and purpose often becomes evident under specific sets of circumstances and events or, especially in the later years, life in general. Sometimes feelings of uselessness contribute to despair and depression. Pondering over one's past may convey feelings of pride or of a seemingly wasted and worthless life. Illness or other misfortunes raise the question, "Why me?" or "Why does God let me live?" There often is a more or less conscious search for both *provisional meanings* of the many events of daily living and the *ultimate meanings* of life in general that they reflect (Missinne, 1990). The need for meaning and purpose relates closely to the deeply ingrained desire to maintain one's personal dignity and self-esteem.

The Need for Love and Relatedness

There is substantial evidence that satisfying relationships with other people are important components of physical and emotional wellness. Sharing companionship, conversation, intimacy, laughter, a hug or caressing touch, and giving oneself to others by work or service help to satisfy this need.

Although love is a stereotypical solution for this need, the kind that is a form of self-interest, "If you satisfy my needs, then I will love you," can harm social relationships and self-concepts. Another form of love is expressed in such statements as "I love you because of who you are/what you have/or what you do." It can impose the burden of needing to deserve or earn the other's love and the fear of losing whatever one is loved *because of.*

A third kind of love is an unconditional *in spite of love* like the *agape* love of God. One is loved simply as she or he is, in spite of faults, habits, bad records, or ignorance, and without any demands or strings attached (Shelly and Fish, 1988):

> Self-pity, depression, insecurity, isolation, desperation and fear are some of the indications of a need for love from oneself, other people and God. Feelings of self-worth, joy, security, belonging, hope and courage are experienced on the other end of the spectrum when the need for love is met. These are the benefits of the *in spite of* kind of love God offers to people when they are going through a crisis. (p. 47)

The Need for Forgiveness

Most of us have experienced failures to live up to our own expectations or our beliefs about the expectations of others for us. We may carry an unresolved guilty conscience or a sense of shame for wrongs done or good deeds not done, even promises made but broken and the "if only" regrets connected with bereavement and other losses. We may regret disobedience to parents or an employer, bear a sense of shame for acts or imaginations of infidelity to a spouse, and realize that we have sinned against God. Feelings of worthlessness, hostility, psychological stress, defensiveness, or paranoia typically result. These can be resolved through accepting the forgiveness of God and of others, an awareness of which seldom occurs without confession.

The Need for Spiritual Integration

Interrelated with all our other human needs is "the need to maintain and to illuminate ourselves beyond our existence . . . through an interaction and exchange that goes beyond biophysical and psychosocial facts. . . . We need to know and to feel ourselves spiritually integrated beyond our own existence into an absolute order of existence, which will help us to be more ourselves and to unfold our existence into the global universe" (Missinne, 1990, p. 147). This need is expressed through the hope for immortality, the desire to be at peace with our own conscience and with God, and requests for God's support in the experiences and trials of life. The solution offered varies from one religious or pseudoreligious group to another. Christians find it in the Bible.

The Need to Cope with Losses

One realistic, although depressing, way to look at the aging process is to identify the losses that are common to the human condition during old age, including one's youthful appearance, adult strength, general healthfulness, and independence. Family members and friends are lost when they die or move away from one's local community. There also is loss of a spouse, possessions, a driver's license, and social roles at work, in the community, in organizations like the church, and in the family. All of these have spiritual as well as economic, psychological, and sociological implications. But even losses can enrich one's life journey, for each provides an opportunity for spiritual growth and development (Sullenger, 1999).

The Need for Freedom to Raise Questions

Some have unresolved doubts about the presence of evil in a universe created by a loving God. Many wonder why God allowed illness, disability, bereavement, financial problems, or other burdens to fall upon them or their family (see Hart, 1994, pp. 91-105). They may be angry with God, then feel guilty about their anger. Some think they have committed an unforgivable sin or that God has forsaken them. Usually, it is cathartic for people to share such questions with a sympathetic listener. Spiritual interventions are especially important as a means of resolving such problems, but dogmatic "preaching" or responding with alarm may do more harm than good.

The Need for Flexibility

Old age is a period of life in which many changes are imposed upon people, despite whether they desire and seek them. Rapid technological change in supermarkets, health care, housing, and transportation are often imposed upon even those who insist they themselves will never change. Whether they formally adjust or merely adapt to the changing world around them and their own new situations, they are in fact changing. Flexibility to do so gently, instead of only when wrenching circumstances are forcefully imposed, is an asset that greatly facilitates life satisfaction. Studies of change in the Bible reveal that rigid inflexibility to imitate the changeless God is not commanded for God's people. Yet, as the familiar hymn says, "Change and decay in all about I see. Oh, Thou who changest not, abide with me."

The Need to Prepare for Dying and Death

Much of this preparation seems purely physical and materialistic. Plans should be made for the disposition of one's possessions. Openness about insurance and other means of covering economic costs is advisable. Health and strength can be improved by appropriate life-styles and spiritual nourishment. Usually, most elders fear the dying process more than death itself, so realistic information is needed about technologies that enable mobility and independence far beyond previous possibilities and about modern medicine to relieve the pain that sometimes accompanies fatal illness. But also old emotional accounts from past mistakes and grudges can be settled.

Spiritual interventions to help dying patients find peace with God and with their survivors can do much to make the anticipated departure from this life less foreboding and to live joyfully even when life is less than perfect. Spirituality can help also to overcome the delusions of immortality that deceive some people, as well as the resistance of family members against helping the older generation prepare for their demise. In addition, Carson (1989, pp. 275-278) has shown how health professionals can serve dying patients wrestling with their fate by asking six brief questions in a personal spiritual survey that probes their perception of God, their belief system, the form their praying usually takes, convictions about the meaning of their own life, thoughts about the "why" of illness and suffering, and thoughts and feelings about their own dying and death.

The Need to Be Useful

This is a form of the need to love others and, in turn, to receive love from others. As Jesus said, "It is more blessed [happiness-conducive] to give than to receive" (Acts 20:35, NIV). Even frail, ill, and disabled persons can still be helpful to their companions and those who serve them in such ways as speaking encouraging words to them in their times of difficulty and grief, thanking them, giving them satisfaction in their service, sharing vignettes of their life story that fit the other's needs, and prayer.

The Need to Be Thankful

Just as a sore toe or thumb tends to catch all of our attention, other burdens and problems of life tend to do the same. Surly pouting and cantankerous griping tend to accumulate, building up like accretions of mud and trash in the delta of a river and making other people avoid the source as much as possible. The increased isolation, in turn, accelerates the vicious circle and aggravates feelings of doom and gloom. The life review can stimulate a more balanced perspective that includes one's happy experiences, profitable accomplishments, and good circumstances. As another old hymn says, "Count your blessings, name them one by one, and it will surprise you what the Lord has done." Again, Scripture and accounts others share in a spiritual group can be a significant source of help.

Numerous Other Spiritual Needs

Numerous other spiritual needs can be and have been identified. Missinne (1990), for example, believes that each human being has the need for biophysical exchange, psychosocial exchange, and spiritual integrated exchange. Koenig (1994, pp. 284-294) lists fourteen spiritual needs, many overlapping with those already discussed. The precise needs of any given individual vary with personal circumstances, background, disposition, and faith orientation, so sensitivity is needed lest friends or professionals impose or create the burden of assumed needs upon everyone. The Bible provides countless passages of comfort, counsel, and help to assist with meeting all human needs. When correctly used, it is a resource of inestimable value, speaking especially to elders with a Jewish or Christian background.

THE SPIRITUAL LIFE REVIEW

"Telling one's story" is a wholesome exercise for almost everyone, whether the audience is oneself alone, family members, a support group, historical archives of an organization or community, or some other focus. Reminiscing helps to integrate one's personality, to discern the directions in which one has been and is going, to sharpen one's purpose for living, to clarify the significance of one's life, and sometimes to change its course (see Georgemiller and Getsinger, 1987). Especially during later adulthood, it helps to answer questions about such matters as how one's life has made a difference to others; why one feels as one does about oneself; whether one's attitudes toward other people and the world are what they ought to be; what one has learned from past accomplishments and experiences; how one has benefited from experiences of injustice, disappointment, and loss; and what is the meaning and significance of one's life.

"Sharing stories has a profound healing effect" (Sullivan, 1993, p. 33), for it helps to integrate the body, mind, and spirit. Hearing the life stories of others usually is fascinating and helpful to the listeners, whether they are the children or grandchildren of the teller or only acquaintances and friends. As Tony Perrino (1997), chaplain for a visiting nurse and hospice association, put it, "I have never known a patient whose personal story wasn't significant" (p. 2). Part of the value of life reviews is that, even for dying persons, ". . . occasionally there's some unfinished business to be dealt with . . . , [so] giving encouragement to take care of such matters is the crucial task of spiritual caregiving" (p. 2).

Especially important to the meaning and purpose-in-life aspects of any life review are its spiritual components. Sharing one's spiritual autobiography with others is a very significant way to clarify one's own spirituality and grow toward spiritual maturity. When done in a sympathetic group, it often awakens disheartened people to the fact that they indeed did make important contributions to their family, workplace, or others in the world, so their life was worthwhile after all. Feedback from hearers also provides help to solve many of life's remaining puzzles, resolve its dilemmas, and explain past or present paradoxes. One of the best published sources, *Telling Your Story, Exploring Your Faith* (Hateley, 1985), is an excellent manual and a major stimulus for some of the following details.

A life review focused around the spiritual aspects of a person's autobiography helps to cope with all spiritual needs. People of faith often have questions about why God allowed certain perplexing events to happen. Why did God sometimes seem to desert them in their times of special need? In current discouraging circumstances, can there be any hope for their future in this life or the next? Openly sharing "the dark night of the soul" (not just the "brightness" of accomplishments and prestige) with sympathetic listeners brings cathartic relief. For believers, the discussion that accompanies baring one's soul can clar-. ify the promises of Scripture and show how God was at work in similar experiences of others. It produces or strengthens the relieving assurance that, despite all that is occurring, God has not abandoned them to their fate, but is still at work in their lives.

Especially when it is written, the spiritual life review passes along one's heritage of faith and spiritual wisdom—a "spiritual bequest"—to family members and friends, potentially contributing to their spiritual development. It is an all too often neglected method by which Christians can "teach and admonish one another" (Colossians 3:16, NIV). Through it they can "Carry each other's burdens, and in this way . . . fulfill the law of Christ" (Galatians 6:2, NIV). It helps both the teller of the life story and the listeners to recognize that "in all things God works for the good of those who love him" (Romans 8:28, NIV).

HOW TO PREPARE
A SPIRITUAL LIFE REVIEW

"Every person is an unfinished story" (Sullivan, 1991, p. 5), but, beyond the ethics of honesty, there is no single "correct" method for preparing and presenting a spiritual autobiography. St. Augustine's *Confessions* and other literary autobiographies are prominent examples. Today life stories often are shared orally or on audiotape or videotape with family members or friends. Many are self-written. Others are tape recorded and then transcribed for use in research, self-help groups, psychological therapy, historical archives, or family histories.

The process of recording or writing a life review can be stimulated by memorabilia such as letters, scrapbooks, photo albums, diaries, household furnishings, travel records, and old financial reports or income tax records. Some prefer to give a chronological record of their personal spiritual history, others one that is focused around major events, while still others comment on emotions and feelings related to life experiences. Conversations with other family members and friends can stimulate the retrospective process and enrich the reminiscences.

Since one's life resembles a story in process, it has no end until death. Some persons continue telling their story by keeping a spiritual journal or diary. In it they record notes on their thoughts, prayers, inspirations, observations, insights, spiritual problems, praises, progress, retrogressions, resolutions, theological revelations, choice Bible verses, and more. These sharpen the awareness that all of life is a school for spiritual development.

The following suggestions to stimulate one's life review overlap with one another conceptually and experientially. Since every person is different, the order of the details can vary, and the stimuli that work for one person may not for another. (Many additional suggestions are found in such resources as Hateley, 1985; Quinnan, 1994; and Sullivan, 1991.)

List Major Turning Points in Life

Beginning at birth, when did major changes occur? Possible turning points include school entries and changes, residential moves, vocational choices, friendships and social relationships, group memberships, engagement, marriage, other family events, selecting or buying a home, job changes, promotions and demotions, investments, child bearing and rearing, children's and grandchildren's experiences, family conflicts and tensions, celebrations, volunteer services, retirement, accidents, and illness. They may be religious events such as baptism, confirmation, conversion, confession, repentance, Bible study, becoming a church member, and serving through religious agencies. The spiritual significance of these may not be apparent on the surface, but try to reconstruct what it seemed to be at the time, whether or not you then realized its spiritual significance. Then reappraise their spiritual impact or importance from your current perspective or from its influence upon subsequent events and spiritual growth.

Describe the Problematic Events, Feelings, and Understandings of Your Life

As you do so, consider both the *explanatory* dimension of the meaning of life (why things were, are, and will be) and its *normative* dimension (how they ought to be). What were your religious doubts and fears during childhood, adolescence, young adulthood, and later periods of life, including now? Did any "tragedies" occur? How did you cope with each? Which ones still bother you? Problem experiences may be awakened by recalling times when you asked yourself, "Why did God allow this to happen?" When and how did you yield to temptations to sin? Did you repent and change your conduct, redefine your thoughts or behavior as not sinful after all, or modify them in some other way as a result of increased understanding and education? When and how did you feel that Satan was tempting you or that God was testing your faith? Who or what helped you to cope with those feelings? How did you react to "church fights," hypocritical behavior, or other tensions in a church or other religious groups?

Count Your Blessings

What has God done for you throughout your life from earliest childhood to the present? Be specific! Include what God enabled you to do on behalf of others, both through ministries and day-to-day life activities. How have God's promises been fulfilled in your life? "Harvesting past experiences" of ways in which God has helped in the sorrows and trials of life, as well as in its joys, is an important source of spiritual strength for each day.

Discern the Spiritual Meanings of Life Events

This may include interpretations of your vocational calling(s), your body as a temple of the Holy Spirit, and spiritual influences upon morality and decision making, plus God's plan for your life, his forgiving grace, divine intervention in life events, how your concept of "God the Father" influenced personal experiences for better or worse, the impact of "stewardship" or other theological doctrines upon your beliefs and behavior, your views of death and the afterlife (including heaven and hell), ways in which you followed or rejected the Lord's leading, how church participation affected your faith positively and negatively, answered and seemingly nonanswered prayers, heroes and other models (biblical, familial, historical, literary, etc.) that influenced your thoughts and actions, and the spiritual (including antispiritual) aspects of the personal philosophy that shapes the meaning and goals of your life. Who or what occupies the central place in your thoughts? in your behavior? in priorities for your use of time?

The Bible can be "both a role model and a motivator for us to re-member, share and interpret our own and each other's stories. . . . The process of life review is greatly impoverished in the absence of the Scriptures and, likewise, the study of the Bible is impoverished in the absence of the process of life review" (Rost, 1998, p. 7).

Plot a Spiritual Lifeline

A spiritual lifeline can be a large graph with columns for each year of your life and rows for rating one's levels of spirituality. It can be di-vided at a middle "neutral" line so you can plot the spiritually positive periods or events above it and the spiritually negative events below. (The strongest effects upon your spirituality will be plotted highest or lowest, that is, farthest above or below the middle neutral position.) This tool can be used for probing existential questions as well as for evaluating spiritual growth (Gross, 1985).

For What Spiritual Legacy
Do You Want to Be Remembered?

Most people give attention during their later years to the legacy of material things they will leave behind. When they move into a smaller residence or retirement community, treasured possessions are passed along to family members or friends. Through estate plan-ning, a will is made to indicate how financial assets and property should be distributed after their demise. Notes are prepared to tell who should receive such personal items as a favorite rocking chair, bedspread, set of dishes, or family heirlooms.

Few, however, give attention to leaving a spiritual legacy, although everyone does just that informally through memories of one's faith or scorn for things of faith and of religious and spiritual experiences that were shared with or observed by others.

The subject of what will be one's spiritual legacy may be disturb-ing to many. Anyone who is reluctant about revealing less than per-fection might be frightened away from such self-evaluations. I once interviewed in depth several persons who were deemed either by their pastors to be the most spiritual members of their congregations or by their friends to be the most spiritual people they knew. Without ex-ception, every one of them said that they had not yet reached 100 percent on an imaginary scale of spiritual well-being; they all were still growing toward that goal.

Yet the question, *For what do I most wish to be remembered spiritually?*, can stimulate spiritual growth during the later years of life. Simply answering it is a spiritual exercise in itself. Then, having answered it, one could make three lists:

1. What have I already done that has contributed to that objective?
2. What am I doing and being now to bring that memory to others?
3. What can I do during the rest of my life to make it more certain that I will attain that goal?

For some, no changes will be needed. For others, this exercise may lead to significant modifications of activities and priorities for behavior.

Share Your Life Review with Others

The benefits of the spiritual life review are greatest when they are shared with others. This can occur in family settings or with individual children, grandchildren, nieces, and nephews. It can occur in group settings such as senior center discussions, presentations at grandparent-grandchild banquets, prayer circles, and religious education classes. The questions that emerge usually stimulate the memory and clarify details, and the comments shared often reveal that "God was at work, after all!"

Most spiritual values that specify right from wrong, good from bad, spiritually edifying from spiritually degenerating, and similar norms are connected with the ethics of one or another particular religious orientation. Sometimes the evaluative guidelines that emerge from one faith tradition clash with those of another, so some persons who hear the life story may feel that incidents reported with praise, or even adoration, really ought to be labeled mistakes. Tolerance for the values of others is essential in order to maintain good relationships with them. This does not require approving their value orientations, and asking questions about the whys and wherefores may be appropriate as a means of understanding and value clarification for both the narrator and listener.

Each faith orientation has its own philosophical and theological principles that provide the normative foundation or validating rationale for spiritual life reviews. The following guidelines for sharing those reviews were developed explicitly for use in the context of Christian biblical values. Nevertheless, secular groups and people with different faith orientations will find that most of the same ethical principles fit their values as well.

GUIDELINES FOR SHARING
SPIRITUAL LIFE REVIEWS

Every group has a stated or implied purpose and other limitations for its gatherings. Therefore each life review *presenter* will be able to share only a few faith stories or highlights of his or her autobiography, ideally with a focus upon incidents and experiences that most closely fit the purpose of the group. Seldom is it wise to narrate or confess wrongdoing or sins that impinge upon the lives of other people.

Sharing spiritual experiences with others contributes to the "deposit of faith"—the record of God's loving care among people still living today. It augments biblical histories of how God can use transformed sinners (like Abraham, Moses, David, and Saints Peter and Paul) to accomplish his purposes. It is a significant means of complying with biblical instructions to encourage each other (e.g., 1 Thessalonians 5:11; Hebrews 3:13; 10:25).

A typical Christian support group gathers specifically to deepen the members' spirituality, help them cope spiritually with life experiences, and increase their understanding of biblical faith. Often a life story can be compared to or linked with one or more Bible passages or characters.

The listeners to life reviews should be as ethical as the tellers. From the perspective of Christian values, the following are ten suggestions for listeners:

1. *Listen attentively.* Hear the unexpressed feelings, both positive and negative, that lie within and beneath the spoken message. Sympathetic listening is a therapeutic act of Christian love.
2. *Do not be judgmental.* No one should be ridiculed or "put down" because of what is shared. Remember that we all have made mistakes and have done foolish things. (See Isaiah 53:6; 64:6; Romans 3:23; etc.) Not only that, even the strongest Christians are still sinners (I John 1:8), so, as Jesus taught, we ought not try to cast

the "speck of sawdust" out of another's eye as if we have no "plank" in our own (Matthew 7:1-5). No person's story is superior to another's, even if some seem more dramatic than others.

3. *Respect confidentiality.* Some aspects of one's life are very intimate. Private information could become a part of destructive gossip. Do not violate the right to privacy by passing along painful or sensitive information.

4. *Allow the expression of feelings,* whether of anger and pain, joy or grief, that often accompanies the sharing of deep-seated memories. The release of pent-up feelings, even to the point of tears, can help to heal wounds, so respond to emotions with love and understanding.

5. *Do not usurp the role of either God or a professional therapist* by trying to give absolute or final solutions for any continuing problems the presenter shares. While one may suggest that the person consider different actions or thought patterns, too much emphasis upon "the solution" can make him or her feel downtrodden, self-conscious, and defensive for not having already done what is proposed. Besides, there may be hidden dimensions not shared with the group that modify the issue.

6. *Allow group members to withhold sharing.* Do not put pressure on anyone who prefers not to share his or her life experiences. Some may wish not to share anything, and all may have experiences that they prefer to confess only to the Lord. While concealment may support an unhealthy repression of some aspects of their memories, this policy makes group sharing truly voluntary, protects against potential gossip, and prevents some persons from dropping out of the group. By staying, the non-presenters benefit from the accounts of others.

7. *Be warmly supportive of all.* Respect even those persons whose lives include bizarre experiences. Follow the example of Jesus who loved and associated intimately with a wide variety of social outcastes.

8. *Encourage the autobiographer.* One possible way to do this is to ask each member of the group to write a one- or two-sentence note with an affirmation, prayer, or Bible reference that the presenter can take home as a tangible reminder of the group's loving support for his or her continuing spiritual growth.

9. *Pray for the presenter.* In Christian groups it is especially pertinent to have one or several members lead in audible prayers of thanks and petition for the person who has so courageously spoken. Later at home the group members also will pray privately for her or him.

10. *Reflect personally upon the shared life experiences.* How do they throw light upon one's own spiritual journey? Private reflection and group discussions can stimulate an answer. Because God often works in ways that seem mysterious to us, and the Zeitgeist or spirit of the age in which we live is antagonistic toward spiritual appreciation, we all need that help.

CONCLUSION

Telling one's life story is, with very few exceptions, a helpful activity for both the narrator and the audience. It is a means for discerning and clarifying the meaning of one's pilgrimage from birth to old age. When it is shared, it becomes a part of the heritage one leaves behind to benefit others. It answers the prayer,

> Even when I am old and gray, do not forsake me, O God,
> till I declare your power to the next generation,
> your might to all who are to come. (Psalm 71:18, NIV)

Developing a spiritual autobiography is a very important tool for self-analysis, constructing a self-image, and sharing one's legacy with descendants and friends. Together with the meditation that accompanies and stimulates it, the spiritual life review nurtures spiritual growth in the later years of life—growth that still is possible when everything else seems disintegrating and fading away.

REFERENCES

Butler, Robert N. (1975). *Why survive? Being old in America.* NY: Harper & Row.

Carson, Verna Benner (1989). *Spiritual dimensions of nursing practice.* Philadelphia: W.B. Saunders Co.

Georgemiller, R.J. and S.H. Getsinger (1987). Reminiscence therapy: Effects on more and less religious elderly. *Journal of Religion and Aging* 4(2):47-58.

Gross, Gregory D. (1985). The spiritual lifeline: An experiential exercise. *Journal of Religion and Aging* 1(3):31-37.

Hart, Thomas (1994). *Hidden spring: The spiritual dimension of therapy.* Mahwah, NJ: Paulist Press.

Hateley, Barbara J. (1985). *Telling your story, exploring your faith: Writing your life history for personal insight and spiritual growth.* St. Louis, MO: CBD Press.

Hendricks, Jon (Ed.) (1999). *The meaning of reminiscence and life review.* Amityville, NY: Baywood Publishing Co.

Ison, Jill (1998). A tapestry of lives. *Aging and Religion* 2(February):1-8.

Kimble, Melvin A. (1995). Pastoral care. In Kimble, Melvin A., Susan H. McFadden, James W. Ellor, and James J. Seeber (Eds.), *Aging, spirituality, and religion: A handbook* (pp. 131-147). Minneapolis, MN: Fortress Press.

Koenig, Harold G. (1994). *Aging and God: Spiritual pathways to mental health in midlife and later years.* Binghamton, NY: The Haworth Press.

Missinne, Leo E. (1990). Christian perspectives on spiritual needs of a human being. In Seeber, James J. (Ed.), *Spiritual maturity in the later years* (pp. 143-152). Binghamton, NY: The Haworth Press.

NIV: *The Holy Bible,* New International Version (1984). Colorado Springs, CO: International Bible Society.

Perrino, Tony (1997). Walking through the valley of the shadow. *Aging & Spirituality* 8(4):1-2, 8.

Quinnan, Edward J. (1994). Life narrative and spiritual journey of elderly male religious. In Thomas, L. Eugene and Susan A. Eisenhandler (Eds.), *Aging and the religious dimension* (pp. 147-165). Westport, CT: Auburn House.

Rost, Robert A. (1998). From life review to sacred remembrance. *Aging and Religion* 2(May):1-12.

Shelly, Judith Allen and Sharon Fish (1988). *Spiritual care: The nurse's role,* Third edition. Downers Grove, IL: InterVarsity Press.

Sullenger, R. Scott (1999). *Losses in later life: A new way of walking with God.* Binghamton, NY: The Haworth Press.

Sullivan, Elaine M. (1993). The importance of the human spirit in self-care for older adults. *Generations* 17(3, Fall):33-36.

Sullivan, Paula Farrell (1991). *The mystery of my story: Autobiographical writing for personal and spiritual development.* Mahwah, NJ: Paulist Press.

Chapter 13

The Role of the Chaplain in Spiritual Care

Nils Friberg

The purpose of this chapter is to describe spiritual care given by chaplains in various institutional gerontological settings, define chaplaincy and spiritual care, delineate the more common patterns of practice in these facilities, and, finally, make recommendations for the future.

VARIETIES OF CHAPLAINS

The origin of the English word, "chaplain," can be traced to the Latin, *cappa* (cloak/cape, in English). Around the eighth century, the French monarch's royal cloak or cape was guarded during battles in a small room or building called a *cappella* (English: chapel). The person who was assigned to guard both the cape and the chapel was called a *cappellanus.* The English word, chaplain, came to us, therefore, from Latin through French. Thus the English word still carries a second "a" in it, even though it is not pronounced. Many English speakers have difficulty remembering to include that letter when they write the word.

The development of the chaplain's role probably began in the Middle Ages with the use of clergy to assist monarchs, bishops, and other high ecclesiastical dignitaries (Cross, 1997). Chaplains gradually came to be employed in schools, colleges, prisons, hospitals, cemeteries, embassies, legations, and consulates abroad (Smith, 1990). Today in England and the United States, as well as in several other countries, all military branches and many hospital and prison systems now include chaplaincy (Cross, 1997). Plummer (1996) described several more recently formulated chaplaincies, including workplace settings, racetracks, airports, police systems, and fire fighting. In terms of U.S. hospitals, many authors trace the earliest clarification of a chaplain's role to the writings of Richard Cabot, a famous medical doctor who had strong religious convictions, and Russell Dicks, a chaplain. Their groundbreaking manual *The Art of Ministering to the Sick* (Cabot and Dicks, 1936), powerfully shaped the pastoral care movement, especially the formation of clinical-pastoral education of chaplains in hospitals (Hollifield, 1983).

Chaplaincy and Nursing Care

Historically, nursing of infirm elderly persons was often carried out in the home by family members, with periodic visits from physicians, nurses, and clergy. Today, the focus has shifted to caring for the infirm outside the home in facilities ranging all the way from assisted living to skilled nursing care. Continuing care facilities also contract to care for retirees all the way through to their death, moving them from one type of facility to progressively more intense nursing care. Many also provide hospice care or contract for it with hospice providers.

Most of these care facilities are for-profit, but the American Association of Homes and Services for the Aged, Washington, DC, counts over 5,000 not-for-profit organizations in its membership. It is important to note, however, that there are cultural differences among Americans regarding nursing home use. African Americans tend to use nursing home facilities less than whites, for example (Wimberly, 1997, p. 161).

Understanding what a chaplain is and does presents a greater challenge than spelling the word or knowing the history. In a nursing home administrators' publication, one chaplain complained that ". . . most people don't understand chaplaincy, i.e., do not know what it really constitutes. . . . Most managers do not realize the tremendous resource they have available in this [chaplaincy] and do not, therefore, know how to tap it" (Vance, 1997, p. 59). To this we add the observation that only those nursing care facilities that have a clear sense of mission for spiritual care are involved today in this effort. However, with ever-tightening budget constraints, even they are encountering difficulty maintaining the level of spiritual care by chaplains that they desire (Cartwright, 1999).

It is difficult to know how many of the estimated 17,000-plus (American Health Care Association, 1999) long-term care facilities in the United States employ fully trained and paid chaplains. Even though many of these facilities were founded by faith communities or by people of faith, it is clear to this observer that a large percentage of facilities do not employ adequately trained chaplains. They often either simply invite residents' ministers to visit, or they leave spiritual care up to an activity or volunteer services director. Spiritual care is then reduced to periodic, friendly support and to the coordination and planning of chapel services led by local clergy or lay people from various congregations. Such services seldom are executed with strategically planned care for the special needs of persons with dementia or such other conditions present in this population as mental status, feelings of grief and loss, or family system issues.

If we add to this picture descriptions of the effects of managed care, frequent health care industry mergers, and the resultant bottom-line orientation for the benefit of stockholders, there is good reason for alarm. One Roman Catholic writer opined: "Mounting shadows darken our calling and threaten to transform healing from a covenant into a business contract. . . . Increasingly, patient comfort and the special needs of the elderly, infirm, or disabled are ignored if they conflict with the calculus of profit" (Kavanaugh, 1998, pp. 37-38).

RESOURCES FOR CHAPLAINCIES

There are some good signs on the horizon, however, since resources for meeting these needs are available, though not as ubiquitous and accessible as we would like.

In over 300 centers around the United States, the Association for Clinical Pastoral Education offers seminarians and pastors specialized training for giving spiritual care in many settings. Students are challenged by supervisors and colleagues in small groups to integrate their personal qualities, their method of ministry, and their theological beliefs for the purposes of attending to the spiritual issues of certain populations. Some centers focus on the populations of nursing care and other long-term care facilities. Examples can found in CPE (clinical pastoral education) programs such as those offered by the HealthEast system and the Good Samaritan Society system, both located in St. Paul, Minnesota. The latter also has a CPE center in a long-term care facility in Kissimmee, Florida. Both HealthEast and Good Samaritan have a reasonably clear mission consciousness concerning adequate chaplaincy for the elderly. They also have structures and personnel in place to carry that mission out.

The Association of Professional Chaplains (APC), formerly known as the College of Chaplains, headquartered in Schaumburg, Illinois, and the National Association of Catholic Chaplains, with its national headquarters in Milwaukee, Wisconsin, are both involved in establishing certification standards for chaplains across the United States. These two organizations, along with others, cooperate in an overarching cooperative entity called the Coalition on Ministry in Specialized Settings (COMISS) and their Joint Commission on Accreditation of Pastoral Services (JCAPS). All of these organizations are currently attempting to implement standards for chaplains in health care settings, under the Joint Commission on Accreditation of Healthcare Organizations (JCAHO). It is hoped that improved delivery of spiritual care through chaplains will result in all kinds of health care settings, including those dedicated to service of the elderly. (A full description of these efforts can be found at the Web site <http://www.comiss.org/jcaps.htm>.)

The executive administrator of the APC informed this author that in 1999 the organization included 340 members who state their specialization as aging/geriatrics/long-term care. With some overlap, there is also a group of 225 members who are specialized hospice chaplains (Schrader, 1999). One can only hope that the numbers of specialized chaplains will grow along with the burgeoning population of elderly. Probably additional hundreds of nursing facility chaplains do not belong to APC.

Theological education has long needed a stronger mission consciousness concerning the aged (Moberg, 1975; Payne and Brewer, 1989a). One professor in a theological seminary that stands out as a leading exception states succinctly: "Course offerings in pastoral care and ministry with the aging in theological education curricula . . . have been conspicuous by their absence" (Kimble, 1995, p. 133).

Such a ministry focus struggles to compete with the pressures from churches for seminarians to take courses in leadership, church planting and vision casting, concerns about reaching youth, and more exciting ministries of crisis, conflict, and evangelism. When listening to young, enthusiastic seminarians report in class on their weekend church ministries, one hears such comments as: "That church is over half white hair—there's no future there!" Ministry to the aged and chaplaincy to institutionalized elderly are seldom on seminarians' priority lists. This in spite of the growing numbers in the sixty-five-plus category.

However, there are encouraging signs on the horizon. Payne and Brewer (1989a, b) brought together reports from seven theological schools in which courses and even specialized degree programs are being offered for ministry to the aging. They also surveyed the course offerings of 113 other accredited seminaries in the United States and found evidence of increasing interest and offerings in this area. It is clear in the light of the need, however, that increased efforts at raising the consciousness of seminary students are necessary.

The American Association of Retired Persons (AARP, 1989) has published guidelines for pastoral care for older persons in long-term care settings. Its small brochure written by an eleven-member committee of eldercare chaplains gives helpful descriptions of chaplaincy and pastoral care:

> The spiritual dimension of an individual is basic to life and identity. Spiritual beliefs and convictions give life meaning. The integration of a person's physical, emotional and spiritual [issues] contributes to a sense of well-being. The chaplain assumes primary responsibility to work with other health care staff to facilitate spiritual support, growth, and development within the health care setting. The chaplain and the comprehensive pastoral care program address spiritual needs in many different ways. (p. 8)

This brochure provides an excellent rationale for chaplaincy services in long-term facilities, mentioning, e.g., that these "residents . . . frequently struggle with issues of loss, grief, chronic illness, and increased dependency, while others [outside the facility] are celebrating the experiences of satisfying family relationships, recovery, and new opportunities" (p. 10). When we add dementia, which is frequently present in these older populations, we easily perceive that being an effective chaplain in such settings requires specialized training and competence (VandeCreek, 1999).

Along with these resources, people entering a ministry of this kind must prepare themselves well in terms of their personal self-care resources, especially their psychosocial and spiritual support systems. While it is true that one receives a great deal from the elderly in these ministry settings, there is a definitely discouraging feature to it because there is no cure for the degenerative features of dementia and other debilitating effects of advanced aging. Facing disability and death on a constant basis can stress the strongest of us. Resistance to the natural tendency toward callousness and depression should not depend solely upon the individual chaplain. Both small group and individual spiritual direction are extremely important for people ministering in such settings. Ongoing supervision for counseling issues is also an important resource for growth and satisfaction in difficult settings.

ETHICAL ISSUES

By definition, most chaplains are assigned to populations with limitations related to their own faith communities and congregations because they are either temporarily or permanently institutionalized or otherwise unable to stay in touch with them. This means that there must be ethical guidelines in place to govern the way that institutional chaplains approach, interact with, and guide those under their care. Chaplains must take care not to violate the residents' sense of personal choice.

Thus, given the "captive audience" status of the bedridden and the psychosocial and spiritual vulnerability of nursing care residents, as well as consideration of their spiritual and cultural diversity, chaplains have a moral obligation to take great care to give priority to each patient's own holistic spectrum of need and faith orientation. With growing populations of immigrants and adherents of religions not previously seen in significant numbers in North America, spiritual care must take diversity and pluralism seriously. Utmost respect for the residents' spiritual and religious histories and orientations is imperative.

Fitchett (1993a) closes his book on spiritual assessment with a helpful chapter entitled "The Spirit of Assessment." He recommends modesty, nonrigidity (which he entitles "playfulness"), personal self-awareness, and cultural self-awareness (pp. 130-131). This spirit entails both self-critique and compassionate valuing of the other. The chaplain needs to develop a sense of holy awe concerning the sacred space of each unique individual. When that attitude is portrayed in a compassionate framework, our ethics will be worked out on a much higher plane.

Although religious bodies historically have actively cared for the poor, the elderly, and the infirm, with the growth in numbers of people over sixty-five during the next half century, there needs to be a renewed call for financial and material resources dedicated to ministries with and for them. This need extends also to the importance of special approaches in prison chaplaincies, for the penal system includes rapidly increasing numbers of elderly prisoners.

ELEMENTS OF "SPIRITUAL CARE": ASSESSMENT/DIAGNOSIS

The term spiritual is very broad in today's usage in the sense that writers seldom refer to theological content, but instead to anthropological, psychological, or interpersonal experience. In addition, because of New Age influences, the term spiritual sometimes carries a pantheistic connotation. For example, some authors refer to spiritual connectedness with each other and the universe or state that there is a divine element in each person. For many Christian, Jewish, and Muslim theologians this definition is problematic, since monotheistic realism posits a Creator who is not to be identified as creation itself, who was before creation and continues to sustain it, and who must not be confused with it.

When such a distinction is made, the use of the term spiritual remains advantageous. Indeed, the term spiritual care has begun to replace pastoral care in hospital nomenclature. The reasoning behind this change seems to be that the word spiritual is broader than any religious group, and it takes into account the diverse pluralism of today's world. It is often pointed out that in the 1990s, baby boomers and busters spoke very positively of their own personal spirituality and still were not clearly connected to any religious group.

A recently issued spiritual care proposal for three new long-term care facilities in the Twin Cities written by the Vice President of Spiritual Care of the HealthEast Care System (St. Paul, Minnesota) nicely illustrates this point:

> The Mission and Philosophy of HealthEast's Senior Services, its facilities and programs, includes a component for the care of the spiritual dimensions of all persons, as integral to a comprehensive approach to care. The Spiritual Care Services of HealthEast are provided with an interfaith perspective and are respectful of the diversity of cultural, spiritual traditions and practices of all. (Hinrichs, 1999b, p. 1)

Some researchers (e.g., VandeCreek et al., 1999) include the functional aspects of religious support, whether intrapersonal or interpersonal, under this broad category of spirituality, but we prefer to follow the lead of Freeman (1998), who defines spirituality as ". . . concern with the transcendent dimensions of life" (p. 7). Fitchett similarly defines spiritual as ". . . the dimension of life that reflects the need to find meaning in existence and in which we respond to the sacred" (1993a, p. 16). Sorajjakool (1998), however, develops a more complete rationale: "If reframing the perception of reality to explain and cope with suffering is the basis of religion, the quest for meaning is therefore closely connected to spirituality. In my personal understanding, spirituality is an attempt to find meaning amid pain, suffering, aging, and dying. For this reason, old age is perhaps the best place to reflect on spirituality" (p. 147).

Work with the elderly demands an adequate diagnostic assessment framework, also known as an assessment matrix, for their spiritual care. Assessment has a definitely broader purpose, however. Ramsey (1998) defines diagnosis in pastoral care as ". . . an evaluative process of discerning the nature of another's difficulty in order to provide an appropriate, restorative response" (p. 6). This implies that such a response is not possible without a good diagnosis or assessment. The issue here is whether or not nursing care facilities of various levels are taking this aspect of spiritual assessment seriously enough. If there is a lack of adequate assessment, there cannot be an adequate response to spiritual needs, and thus the residents will have a lower quality of life. This, in turn, may result in higher mortality and morbidity, creating greater costs for both the facility and ultimately the taxpayer.

Fitchett (1993a, b) has done a great deal for the field in regard to defining and describing this process. He equates diagnosis with assessment. "Assessment is both a statement of a perception and a process of information gathering and interpreting. I use the term assessment as a noun and a verb. Because it is both process and content, it is inherently a dynamic concept" (1993a, p. 17).

Fitchett adds that assessment has both descriptive and normative aspects. Thus, we are finding out what is, then comparing it to what ought to be. In terms of responding to the aging and elderly, we must often temper the "ought" since the aging process leaves us with very limited opportunity to reverse its effects. However, since we have evidence that religious coping helps the elderly, there is reason to look for possible improvements in their lives (Koenig, Smiley, and Gonzales, 1988).

To place spiritual assessment within a larger holistic framework, Fitchett places the spiritual dimension of assessment alongside of six others: medical, psychological, psychosocial, family systems, ethnic and cultural, and societal. When we have taken all those areas of his "7 ×7 model" into consideration in our approach to understanding an elderly resident, then we may proceed to analyze the seven dimensions of the spiritual life, which Fitchett names as: (1) beliefs and meaning, (2) vocation and consequences, (3) experience and emotion, (4) courage and growth, (5) ritual and practice, (6) community, and (7) authority and guidance (1993a, p. 42).

For the individual involved in patient care of the elderly, this model may appear to be too abstract, or especially too complex for practical application. Many long-term care facilities simply ask either the new resident or family members to fill out a small religious census card, stating religious preference, indications of clergy or contact with a local faith community, and statements on the desire to attend chapel, receive communion, and have chaplaincy visits or lay visits. More thorough evaluations of the residents' spiritual needs are made only if staff picks up evidence of special needs, such as difficulty adapting to the facility, tensions with a roommate(s), expressions of doubt, fear or discouragement, family struggles, or statements about dying. These people are then referred to the chaplain or to their own clergy, and perhaps to social services as well. (The probable pattern in many facilities is to not bother with any assessment whatsoever.)

Evidence indicates that chaplains can significantly enhance a resident's experience in a nursing care facility (Koenig, 1994, p. 307; Simmons, 1991). Through the use of prayer, personal counseling, teaching patients prayer, and worship services that include the sacraments, adjustment problems can be reduced for those who are experiencing stressful transitions.

Fitchett's model does provide an overview for analysis that is quite helpful, since it asks the staff person to look at the big picture, and helps the chaplain to examine in more thorough ways the various aspects of spiritual care that a particular resident may need. Caregiver strategy can be only as good as the underlying rationale that supports and informs it.

PRACTICAL ISSUES

This writer held several interviews with various long-term care facility chaplains to prepare for writing this chapter (Sartain, 1999; Cartwright, 1999; Hinrichs, 1999c). A major concern that arose in those interviews stems from the tendency for chaplains to be drawn away from their central focus of spiritual care into administrative and committee work that is only peripheral to their central task. If we define spiritual in such a way as to eliminate the practical, we err to one extreme. If we include too many tangential tasks, we err to the other.

Let's take an example. An attractive philosophy for long-term facilities that is growing in influence and acceptance is the "Eden Alternative," a movement founded in Sherburne, New York, by William H. Thomas and his wife, Judy Meyers Thomas. Briefly stated, their main concern is to reduce the loneliness, helplessness, and boredom of life in long-term care facilities. To accomplish this they introduce such elements as children's visits, pets, plants, multitask staffing, and decision-making input from both staff and residents. They create ways for the elderly to relate better to others, to find usefulness, and to gain empowerment of self. By their own testimony, it takes an estimated three to five years to manage the transition from more traditional approaches to the Eden Alternative, but by 1996 nearly 150 facilities around the country had already moved far enough along to be included in the list of certified residences (Thomas, 1996).

In terms of spiritual care by and with chaplains, the Eden Alternative presents an attractive and illustrative challenge. Loneliness, helplessness, and boredom are foundationally spiritual issues, but they also have quite practical and material ramifications. The concrete ways in which elders are involved in care either positively or negatively influence loneliness, helplessness, and boredom. Since administrators who are open to making such radical changes in their programming and staff orientation might also be open to considering how spiritual life can be enhanced, an integrated approach with chaplaincy and spiritual care could well be implemented.

Judy Meyers Thomas (1999) shared a story that illustrates how a social worker decided to invite a resident to help her reach out to a dying woman who was already the resident's friend. Even though the resident had some early signs of dementia, she rose to the occasion when invited, and gave significant spiritual support to the dying woman. Afterward she shared with the social worker that she was glad she had the opportunity to contribute so significantly to the last moments of her friend's life.

Chaplains could likewise involve residents in appropriate levels of caring spiritually for others, even as they find encouragement from caring for a pet in their room. Well-trained chaplains who have opportunities such as this would certainly want to have a vision that goes beyond dealing with loneliness, helplessness, and boredom. However, the concreteness and immediacy of such practical goals do fit well into most philosophies of spiritual care. The challenge is simply to bring the two strategically together.

Chaplain/Resident Ratios

The two corporate chaplaincy directors this author interviewed have set up ratio standards for their facilities. They establish one full-time equivalency chaplain to every 300 (i.e., 1:300) residents in independent living, 1:200 in assisted living, 1:150 in intermediate care, and 1:75 in skilled care (Hinrichs, 1999a). To amplify coverage, they involve volunteers, eucharistic ministers, diaconal programs, seminary students on practicum assignments, and CPE residents.

Chaplains are used to educate staff people about spiritual care, as well as local clergy and lay ministers who volunteer service in their facilities. Staff members are taught how to recognize and react to needs for referral to chaplains. Chaplains are often involved with ethical decision committees and employee support functions as well, with the express understanding that staff members sometimes need support, guidance, and encouragement in their own lives.

CONCLUSIONS AND RECOMMENDATIONS

With the rise in numbers of elderly in institutions over the next few decades, the needs and opportunities for chaplaincy, spiritual assessment, and effective response are significant. Care facilities may have been shortsighted concerning the cost advantages such care could bring them, to say nothing of the improved quality of life, lowered morbidity and mortality, and decreased staff turnover that would result from such improvements. Theological educators and denominational and faith-community leaders need to reexamine their allocation of resources for this population. People going into ministry need to consider spiritual care of the elderly as an important aspect of their vocational choice. Legislators and health maintenance organizations need to examine how to implement laws and guidelines for the care of the elderly that will remove the financial barriers against providing genuinely holistic care. Eventually this issue becomes a personal one for every one of us. However, the political and business issues present us with a societal and ethical concern of high priority.

REFERENCES

AARP (1989). *Guidelines for pastoral care of older persons in long-term care settings.* Washington, DC: American Association of Retired Persons Pamphlet PF4295(289).

American Health Care Association (1999). R-11: Total and average number of nursing facility residents and average ADL dependence by state. Accessed from World Wide Web, <http://www.ahca.org/research/r11/htm> August 11.

Cabot, Richard and Russell Dicks (1936). *The art of ministering to the sick.* New York: Macmillan.

Cartwright, Scott (1999). Chaplain, White Bear Lake, Minnesota, Care Center. Personal Communication, September 8.

Coalition on Ministry in Specialized Settings (1999). <http://www.comiss.org/jcaps.htm> accessed on the World Wide Web on September 2, 1999.

Cross, Frank L. (1997). "Chaplain," and "Chapel," in *The Oxford dictionary of the Christian church* (pp. 319-320). New York: Oxford University Press.

Fitchett, George (1993a). *Assessing spiritual needs: A guide for caregivers.* Minneapolis, MN: Augsburg Press.

Fitchett, George (1993b). *Spiritual assessment in pastoral care: A guide to selected resources.* Decatur, GA: Journal of Pastoral Care Publications.

Freeman, Arthur (1998). Spirituality, well-being and ministry. *The Journal of Pastoral Care* 52(1):7-18.

Hinrichs, Scott (1999a). "Spiritual care proposal: HealthEast senior care" (unpublished document). St. Paul, MN: HealthEast Senior Services.

Hinrichs, Scott (1999b). "Standards for spiritual care system" (unpublished document). St. Paul, MN: HealthEast Senior Services.

Hinrichs, Scott (1999c). Vice President for Pastoral Care, HealthEast, St. Paul, MN. Interview, August 10.

Hollifield, E. Brooks (1983). *A history of pastoral care in America.* Nashville, TN: Abingdon Press.

Kavanaugh, John F. (1998). Capitalism's cost to care. *America* 178(8):37-38.

Kimble, Melvin (1995). Pastoral care. In Kimble, Melvin, S. H. McFadden, J. W. Ellor, and J. J. Seeber (Eds.), *Aging, spirituality and religion* (pp. 131-147). Minneapolis, MN: Fortress Press.

Koenig, Harold G. (1994). *Aging and God: Spiritual pathways to mental health in midlife and later years.* Binghamton, NY: The Haworth Press.

Koenig, Harold G., Mona Smiley, and Jo Ann Ploch Gonzales (1988). *Religion, health and aging: A review and theoretical integration.* Westport, CT: Greenwood Press.

Moberg, David O. (1975). Needs felt by the clergy for ministries to the aging. *The Gerontologist* 15(2):170-175.

Payne, Barbara and Earl D. C. Brewer (Eds.). (1989a). *Gerontology in theological education.* Binghamton, NY: The Haworth Press.

Payne, Barbara and Earl D. C. Brewer (Eds.). (1989b). *Gerontology in theological education: Local program development.* Binghamton, NY: The Haworth Press.

Plummer, David B. (1996). Chaplaincy: The greatest story never told. *The Journal of Pastoral Care* 50(1):1-12.

Ramsey, Nancy J. (1998). *Pastoral diagnosis: A resource for ministries of care and counseling.* Minneapolis, MN: Fortress Press.

Sartain, Gary (1999). Director of Spiritual Care, The Evangelical Lutheran Good Samaritan Society. Personal communication, August 13.

Schrader, Jo (1999). Executive Administrator, Association of Professional Chaplains. Schaumburg, IL. Personal communication, September 2.

Simmons, Henry C. (1991). Teach us to pray: Pastoral care of the nursing home resident. *The Journal of Pastoral Care* 45(2):169-175.

Smith, K.W. (1990). Chaplain/chaplaincy. In Rodney Hunter (Ed.), *The dictionary of pastoral care and counseling* (p. 136). Nashville, TN: Abingdon Press.

Sorajjakool, Siroj (1998). Gerontology, spirituality, and religion. *The Journal of Pastoral Care* 52(2):147-156.

Thomas, Judy Meyers (1999). Eden Miracle. *Eden Talks.* E-mailed copy, dated September 3.

Thomas, William H. (1996). *Life worth living: How someone you love can still enjoy life in a nursing home—The Eden Alternative in action.* Acton, MA: VanderWyk and Burnham.

Vance, Russell E., III (1997). The role of the chaplain: This spirited counselor may have more to offer than you realize. (Chaplains in Long-term Facilities). *Nursing Homes* 46(8):59-61.

VandeCreek, Larry (Ed.) (1999). *Spiritual care for persons with dementia: Fundamentals for pastoral practice.* Binghamton, NY: The Haworth Press.

VandeCreek, Larry, Kenneth Pargament, Timothy Belavich, Brenda Cowell, and Lisa Friedel (1999). The unique benefits of religious support during cardiac bypass surgery. *The Journal of Pastoral Care* 53(1):19-29.

Wimberly, Anne Streaty. (1997). *Honoring African-American elders.* San Francisco, CA: Jossey-Bass.

POLICY IMPLICATIONS
AND PRIORITIES FOR THE FUTURE

National policy in the United States generally ignores spirituality. This may be mainly a result of its close connections with religion, narrow interpretations of the separation of church and state, and the ever-increasing religious pluralism of the population. In this section, we shall see that, in spite of this, the White House Conferences on Aging have made many proposals related to the spiritual needs of older people, a few of which have culminated in tangible action.

Throughout this book a basic theme has been the need for better knowledge and understanding of human spirituality, as well as for methods by which to evaluate the programs, projects, professional services, and ministries intended to enhance it. Whatever the precise methodologies used for such research and assessments and wherever their settings, many general principles for improving its quality can help to assure honesty and integrity in the process.

Finally, some of the continuing challenges related to spirituality that can help to beneficially orient much of our behavior, organizations, research, and professional life are mentioned. The readings recommended for further study will also contribute to the goal of expanding one's understanding of spirituality and aging.

Chapter 14

Toward Better Care: Connecting Spirituality to the Long-Term Needs of Elders

Stephanie Sue Stein

Today, the long-term care funding policies in the United States guarantee that nursing home care will be the only long-term care option of most frail elders. Despite years of increased regulation, scandal after scandal describing inhumane care is reported in our nation's newspapers. Despite efforts to reform the states' long-term care systems to provide older people choice and dignity and to measure quality of care, most of our nation's elders fear the places where they may be forced to spend their last days.

What is missing? The universal recognition that older persons are not disease or frailty or need alone, but also spirit, and with it the public policy recognition that spirit must be nurtured, honored, and protected for all of life.

But can public policy be formulated to address spirituality, and can policymakers agree on what it means? Do any practitioners of long-term care recognize such spiritual matters, and are they making a difference?

Public policy on aging has been partially formulated in this country since 1961 through White House Conferences on Aging. Reports and recommendations from them are available to those who craft and operate long-term care systems.

This chapter first examines the history of public policy development in spirituality and aging by examining the recommendations of the 1961 to 1995 White House Conferences on Aging (WHCA, 1961; 1971a, b; 1981; 1995a, b). Next the chapter summarizes the history and current state of long-term care policy in the United States. The connections and disconnections between spirituality and long-term care are discussed, and, finally, some model programs are briefly mentioned.

WHITE HOUSE CONFERENCES ON AGING

Thousands of people gathered four times in the twentieth century to craft an Aging Agenda for America. Each of these gatherings, the White House Conferences on Aging, "has had a profound impact on aging policies in this country" (WHCA, 1996, p. 137).

The 1961 White House Conference on Aging spurred the legislation that enacted Medicare and Medicaid. It also led to passage of the Older Americans Act of 1965 and to the creation of aging units or offices in all state governments.

The 1971 White House Conference on Aging recommendations were extraordinarily effective. These recommendations resulted in: (1) Cost of Living Adjustments to Social Security, (2) the Supplemental Security Income (SSI) program, (3) the Elderly Nutrition Program, (4) the House Select Committee on Aging, and (5) the Federal Council on the Aging.

The 1981 White House Conference on Aging was rife with political battles over control, but it led to the 1983 Social Security reforms that averted a crisis involving the solvency of Social Security.

The 1995 White House Conference on Aging spurred a national debate, still raging, over the future of Social Security, Medicare, Medicaid, and the Older Americans Act. The delegates found it necessary to issue strong statements about these bedrock programs. Recommendations still awaiting legislative action include national policies concerning long-term care, Alzheimer's research, and caregiver support.

Public policy recommendations concerning spiritual well-being are contained in each of the four White House Conference on Aging final reports. In three of the four conferences, spiritual well-being had its own content, discussion, and report area. Only at the 1981 White House Conference on Aging were spiritual well-being recommendations and issues interspersed among other issue areas.

The 1961 White House Conference on Aging

The 1961 White House Conference on Aging made fifteen recommendations under the topic of spiritual well-being. The recommendations are heavily weighted toward participatory membership in religious congregations (7 of 15). The other areas addressed are nonmember activities (1), service activities (5), and attitudes toward aging (2).

The participatory membership recommendations admonish congregations to recognize and seek out their older members. They ask congregations to provide meaningful roles for elders and to remove barriers that prevent elders from fulfilling those roles. They recommend providing transportation so elders can attend church and a special dues structure in religious institutions so that elders can continue to contribute. They also recommend outreach and personal ministry to homebound and institutionalized members, using media such as radio, television, and tape recordings.

The next recommendation bridges the gap between congregation-directed action and social- or public-directed action by asking religious communities to reach out and provide programs and opportunities to nonmembers living in their neighborhoods.

The five actions recommended under service activities ask congregations to become involved with and influence the public life of older persons by

1. operating denominational services and facilities;
2. offering church-based programs of counseling and psychotherapy;
3. using their facilities as neighborhood service centers;
4. watchdogging government services to make sure they are operated "in a manner consonant with the nature and dignity of man and the sanctity of existence" (*Inventory of Recommendations,* No. 42, 1971); and
5. working for legislation concerned with retirement and labor practices that would help older persons assume new roles.

The final recommendations, those on attitudes toward aging, ask that the lives, roles, and worth of older persons be celebrated as having intrinsic value and that congregations take the lead in this education and promulgation of thought.

All of the 1961 White House Conference on Aging recommendations are directed at congregational or religious action. It is clear that the delegates recognized the religious community's role in operating services, affecting policy, and championing the lives and spirits of older persons in the public arena. The delegates offered *no* resolutions outlining the government's role in promoting, protecting, or recognizing spiritual well-being in aging persons.

The 1971 White House Conference on Aging

The 1971 White House Conference on Aging's recommendations on spiritual well-being are prefaced by a preamble that first defines spiritual well-being as those aspects of life ". . . pertaining to man's inner resources, especially his ultimate concern, the basic value around which all other values are focused, the central philosophy of life—whether religious, anti-religious or non-religious—which guides a person's conduct, the supernatural and non-material dimensions of human nature" (Moberg, 1971, p. 3). The preamble then clearly and purposefully moves the discussion of responsibility for spiritual well-being from the private to the public sector by stating, "Whether it be the concerns for education, employment, health, housing, income, nutrition, retirement roles, or transportation, a proper solution involves personal identification, social acceptance, and human dignity. These come fully only when man has wholesome relationships with fellowman and God" (*Toward a National Policy,* Volume II, p. 58). In other words, good public policy comes only with attendant spiritual well-being.

There are fourteen policy recommendations from the section on spiritual well-being of the 1971 White House Conference on Aging Final Report. The first six are direct government-driven policy items. The other eight are directed at religious bodies (note the change from the 1961 term—congregations).

The government is asked to

1. cooperate with religious agencies to meet the spiritual needs of the elderly;
2. cooperate with religious organizations to provide research and education about the spiritual needs of the elderly;
3. provide money for training clergy and other professionals to help meet the spiritual needs of the elderly;
4. provide for and pay for chaplaincy services in all institutional settings, and to regulate this through licensing;
5. evaluate all publicly funded programs to determine those programs' effects on the spiritual well-being of the elderly they serve; and
6. ensure that all elders receive information of benefit to them, especially from the Social Security Administration.

Religious bodies are asked to

1. serve elders in conjunction with people of all ages;
2. take religious programming and consultation to homes of shut-ins;
3. be concerned with spiritual, personal, and social needs;
4. refer elders to appropriate services;
5. advocate for the needs of elders;
6. protect the rights of elders;
7. develop interfaith community programs; and
8. affirm reverence for life and the right to die with dignity.

All fourteen recommendations affirm the importance of partnership between the public and religious sectors. They move responsibility for the spiritual well-being of older persons out of an exclusively church domain into one shared with elected officials and administrators. They clearly note that spiritual well-being is intrinsic to the entire fabric of the aging life.

The 1981 White House Conference on Aging

The 1981 White House Conference on Aging had 4,000 delegates and promulgated 668 recommendations, with no specific section on spiritual well-being. An investigation of all of the recommendations uncovers twelve that mention spiritual well-being, spirituality, religion, or the role of the religious community. They are attached to or inserted into broader categories. The categories and their recommendations are as follows.

Older Americans As a Continuing Resource

Recommendation 80. Information should be collected on the needs of the "7 million Euro-Americans" (American citizens born in Europe) who have diverse cultures and religious heritages, in order that they might have fruitful lives.

Promotion and Maintenance of Wellness

Recommendation 108. To promote and maintain a sense of well-being among seniors, mental and spiritual, as well as physical, health should be specifically included in all concerns (a holistic approach).

Options for Long-Term Care

Recommendation 180. That the Congress establish a volunteer ombudsman program in order that the spiritual well-being of the patient receiving the attention improves relations with staff and patient's family.

Family and Community Support Systems

Recommendation 219. (The most inclusive recommendation.) Reaffirms the 1971 White House Conference on Aging's recognition of spiritual well-being as a major concern, adopts the National Interfaith Coalition on Aging (NICA) definition of spiritual well-being, calls for national policy to include the spiritual well-being dimension, calls for a Blue Ribbon panel to develop strategies to originate and disseminate spiritual well-being directions into all sectors and, finally, recommends that "All legislative and program language must include the spiritual well-being dimension" (from Committee 7, p. 3).

Recommendation 220. An integrated system of services with religious groups sharing responsibility for implementation with the public and private sectors.

Conditions for Continuing Community Participation

Recommendation 373. Religious groups should not be prohibited from being full partners in services due to constitutional separation of church and state.

Recommendation 374. NICA should establish training programs which would be disseminated by the government to train professionals.

Recommendation 375. Government should work with NICA and the National Council of Churches to publicize and disseminate lists of services offered by religious institutions.

Recommendation 376. Calls on secular and religious organizations to develop services that meet holistic needs of older people.

Private Sector: Roles, Structures, Opportunities

Recommendation 478. Brings to the attention of the Aging Network benefits of working with religious organizations and urges religious organizations to be more involved with needs of older persons.

Recommendation 479. Government should continue funding religious organizations that provide social services at the same level, and local governments should be mandated to fund religious organizations rather than start new ones.

Research

Recommendation 609. Federally funded research should examine the effects of religious involvement and spiritual well-being on the longevity and quality of life of older persons (note: this research again references "Euro-Americans") (WHCA,1981, p. 5).

These recommendations are soft, scattered, and, for the most part, neither government nor religious institution based. They call for cooperation, information sharing, and dissemination. They add little to the base established in 1961 and 1971.

The 1995 White House Conference on Aging

The 1995 White House Conference on Aging did have a spiritual well-being section, but it added "Ethics, Values, and Roles" to the title. Whereas two recommendations were proposed to the delegates, only one—encouraging the development and ensuring the implementation of advance directives—was passed. The second resolution—meeting the spiritual needs of older persons—which included the call for a national conference on "The Third Age and Spiritual Well-Being in the 21st Century" (WHCA, 1995a, p. 8), did not receive sufficient delegate votes.

Summary

The 1961 White House Conference on Aging focused on congregational responsibility. The 1971 WHCA called for both government action and action from religious communities. NICA, founded in 1972, was one of its direct results. The 1981 WHCA called for cooperation, study, and dissemination, and the 1995 White House Conference on Aging called only for the use of Advance Directives. Political agendas shaped each of these formal reports. However, in 1971 social programs were new, exciting, and growing. By 1995 even Social Security and Medicare were under attack. Rather than create and build, the delegates chose to defend and protect.

After almost four decades, is the spirituality, spiritual well-being, and wholeness of life protected in public policy and aging? Are four decades of thought and action incorporated into the programs that serve older people? Social Security, Medicare, and the Older Americans Act are the fundamental programs that philosophically reflect a basic floor of services and structures for older persons in their inception and amendments.

HISTORICAL TRENDS

More difficult to examine, but perhaps most important to understand, are public policies in long-term care. Do the manifestations of long-term care policies bear witness to spiritual well-being, ". . . the affirmation of life in a relationship with God, self, community, and environment that nurtures and celebrates wholeness" (National Interfaith Coalition on Aging, 1975; see Ellor 1997) of older persons? Further, is there evidence that the religious community plays a role in monitoring or advancing the spiritual well-being of older persons in long-term care, or that government laws, monitoring, or regulations include spiritual well-being in policy?

"Long-term care includes a broad range of services needed by people with chronic illness or disabling conditions over a long period of time" (Stone, 1999, p. 2). Long-term care services are generally described as assistance with activities of daily living—"getting in and out of bed, toileting, bathing, dressing, and eating" or the instrumental activities of daily living—"taking medications, preparing meals, financial management, doing light housework and other chores, being able to get in and out of the house, using the telephone and so on" (Holstein and Cole, 1996, p. 5). Although people age sixty-five and over comprised only 57 percent of the 12.8 million Americans with long-term care needs in 1995 (Stone, 1999), as both individuals and society as a whole age, it is the elderly who must be the most concerned about their long-term care needs.

Long-term care can be, and is, provided in a multitude of settings and by different levels of care providers. It can be provided in private homes and apartments; in congregate and assisted living settings; in continuing care retirement communities; and in skilled nursing facilities. According to a General Accounting Office Report in 1994, only 22 percent of the elderly population who needed long-term care resided in nursing homes. The remaining 78 percent received long-term care in home and community settings (Holstein and Cole, 1996). Furthermore, although trained professionals (nurses, home health aides, therapists, etc.) provide most long-term care in institutional settings and through home health agencies, "80 percent of disabled older adults living in the community received unpaid assistance from family and others" (Stone, 1999, p. 2).

Over $100 billion was spent on long-term care in the United States in 1995, with 72 percent spent on nursing home care and 28 percent on home care (Holstein and Cole, 1996). Long-term care is now a catch-all term for dozens of services provided and paid for by many programs, and by older people and their families. How did this system—or nonsystem—evolve, and who was involved in its formation?

Holstein and Cole (1996) trace the evolution of long-term care in America through several statges. A summary of their findings follows.

From the colonial period to the 1820s, families provided virtually all care for poor and infirm elders (Holstein and Cole, 1996). Those too poor or without families depended on care provided by the local community. A shared moral and religious bond in this post-industrial time recognized a communal need for help for the poor. Older people without financial and family support were not treated differently from other poor people; they were part of the community and thus taken care of. This period is often categorized as "outdoor" or noninstitutional relief.

The next period, 1820-1865, saw both the philosophy and the treatment of poverty change to what is known as "indoor" or institutional relief. This period saw the growth of almshouses to house poor persons whom society deemed responsible for their fate and unworthy of humane treatment. These almshouses were not acceptable to *worthy* older Americans (white and Protestant). So homes for the *worthy* respectable persons, mostly women, were founded by religious societies and by local governments. Benevolent societies to provide relief to black Americans were also formed, mainly in the African Methodist Episcopal Church.

From 1865 to 1935, "the changes that occurred had momentous consequences for the development of modern long-term care" (Holstein and Cole, 1996, p. 25). First, due to reforms for other poor persons (children, etc.), almshouses became primarily homes for the poor aged. Second, conditions in almshouses were so deplorable that social reformers deemed them inappropriate for the *worthy aged*. Third, old age was described in terms of inevitable pathology, and institutions were regarded as the appropriate place for care. Fourth, African Americans, who did not have access to either almshouses or health care, formed their own institutions and society. Fifth, religious and cultural institutions founded their own homes in great numbers and added nursing staff. Finally, physicians realized the need for home care for chronically ill people, but no public financing mechanism existed to pay for it. (Tuberculosis sanatoriums were nongovernment organizations supported by contributions from various religious groups.)

"From the 1930s to the 1960s six critical factors shaped the emergence of modern long-term care" (Holstein and Cole, 1996, p. 33). First, Social Security gave older persons some income with which to purchase services. Second, Social Security payments were extended to persons living in institutions, thus shifting the government's burden for payment. Third, two government construction loan programs, the Hill-Burton Act and the Small Business Administration, helped nursing homes proliferate. Fourth, the federal Kerr-Mills program provided federal participation in medical care to poor elders. Fifth, nursing homes joined together to form a strong lobby, the American Association of Nursing Homes. Sixth, the federal government began to set standards for nursing home care.

Holstein and Cole (1996) refer to the period between 1965 and the present as "the Era of Medicare and Medicaid" (p. 39). During this period, homecare was formalized in policy as a substitute for hospital care, not as an alternative to institutional care for people with chronic conditions. Medicare first financed nursing homes but, as costs escalated, their funds soon became restricted to recuperative care. Medicaid, which provided medical coverage for poor persons, soon became the largest source of government payment for institutional care.

> In sum, roughly from 1935 to 1975, the development of nursing homes occurred almost by chance.... For the past twenty years, nursing homes have been the subject of sustained debate and study. (Holstein and Cole, 1996, p. 41)

Although nursing home care remains the most available and highest funded long-term care system, other alternatives are available but woefully underfunded. The most widely used funding source for the home and community based long-term care system is Medicaid Waivers obtained through state governments. Unlike nursing home care, however, waivers are not entitlement programs under Medicaid, and each state chooses how many waiver slots to fund or match with state dollars. "A number of states have demonstrated that a state's long-term care system can be transformed from an almost total dependence on nursing home care to a more comprehensive system of care options" (Coleman, 1996, p. ii).

Older people, when asked, overwhelmingly prefer to live in the community as long as possible (Families USA Foundation, 1993).

Yet home- and community-based Medicaid Waivers have not grown enough to meet the need.

Bruce Vladek, former director of the Health Care Financing Administration, in a speech to the annual meeting of the American Association on Aging on March 16, 1998, in San Francisco, calls this a "public policy stasis" (Vladek, 1998, p. 25). Vladek speculated that states have not fully developed these options because

1. they fear that home and community-based care expansion will increase long-term care spending,
2. there is an absence of solid data on home and community-based programs, and
3. there is no organized effort of elderly advocacy to demand change.

But Larry Polivka (1998), Director of Gerontology at the Florida Policy Exchange Center on Aging, argues that the real reason we have no comprehensive home and community-based system in the United States is the lack of "a moral vision which is critical to creating a political environment that is responsive to the results of research . . . a moral vision to guide the transformation of long-term care for the elderly from a system dominated by institutional care to one characterized by a range of home and community-based options and far more under the control of the frail elderly and their caregivers" (p. 4). Long-term care public policy, both historically and today, is dominated by nursing home care. Nursing home care, by its very nature, removes control and autonomy from the hands and minds and spirits of elders.

Polivka further states, "I don't think we can neatly separate long-term care research from the ethics and politics of long-term care; they are dialectically related. Research results can be used to help formulate an ethic for long-term care which is based on a moral vision designed to resist tendencies to devalue the elderly" (Polivka, 1998, p. 4). Yet there is little doubt that public policy decisions support nursing home care as the only long-term care choice for older persons who cannot afford alternative care in the community.

Spirituality in Long-Term Care

Continuing evidence indicates that nursing home care does not measure up on the enhancement of spiritual well-being, especially as it relates to the environment. There have been many attempts to enhance and improve life in long-term care settings. The proponents of those changes use phrases and words that are strangely similar to the NICA definition of spiritual well-being.

In the fall 1998 edition of *Critical Issues in Aging,* several authors comment on "Getting Serious About Life in Nursing Homes." Kane (1998) writes, "Quality of life is a summary of everything we care about . . . dignity, privacy, a sense of identity, continuity with one's previous life, a sense of meaning, fulfillment, meaningful relationships and social participation, the chance to make a contribution, spiritual well-being, control and choice over one's life" (p. 51). In order to measure quality, she suggests asking residents if they have these things.

Bill Thomas (Kane, 1998), founder of the Eden Alternative, says, "Quality of life is well-being. It is living a life that is full and fully human. The problem with quality of life in long-term care, whether it's assisted living or nursing homes or whatever, is emptiness" (p. 52).

The spiritual challenges of nursing home care are best laid out by Friedman (1995) who states, "Nursing home residents confront critical spiritual challenges, including empty and burdensome time, meaninglessness, and disconnection" (pp. 362-365). He further summarizes these spiritual challenges:

1. Time in an institution is made routine and limited due to staffing schedules.
2. Time is empty—there is a great deal of waiting and a lack of meaningful structure.
3. There is no reality but "now." No one is around who shares the past or who offers hope for the future.
4. Life has no meaning; residents are powerless to control their environment.
5. Residents are disconnected—from the past, from home, from community.

Friedman then suggests some ways that religious life can help nursing home residents:

1. Using religious ritual and adding meaning to every day, each as a part of a sacred whole. Ritual not only connects a person to the past and what he/she celebrated, but also to a future where the rituals will continue.

2. Using religious worship that can be customized so that residents can and must take part gives purpose to their attending.
3. Connecting to the outside faith community through the sameness of worship.
4. Providing a real link to God's care. (pp. 365-368)

Friedman also suggests practical considerations for religious life in nursing homes, such as working out good timing, making sure the rooms and equipment are accessible to frail elders, finding ways for everyone to participate, and involving families and staff. He concludes, "Religious life holds the promise of celebration, meaning and connection to those who will end their life in nursing homes" (p. 372).

Elders in the community, no matter how well served or how determined they are to exercise their autonomy, can suffer from spiritual isolation. Probably the most successful organized effort to link church-sponsored volunteers within the community is the National Federation of Interfaith Caregivers. There are hundreds of interfaith caregiving programs throughout the United States. They all attempt to reach out to the frail elderly and their caregivers and support them through the services of the interfaith community. But long-term care for most elders still means nursing home care.

MODEL PROGRAMS

The most promising models for change are being developed and disseminated by four groups of nursing home operators who are dubbed "pioneers." In the Final Report of the Meeting of Pioneers in Nursing Home Culture Change (Fagan, Burger, and Williams, 1997), the philosophies and strategies of these pioneers are outlined. "Pioneers value and respect residents and staff by . . . seeking to respond to spirit as well as mind and body needs" (p. 28).

These pioneers are about the business of changing nursing home culture, a culture they recognize as being "destructive to health and well-being" and aiming instead to create a culture that "supports life-giving daily experience" (Fagan, Burger, and Williams, 1997, p. 35). The pioneer movements are summarized as follows:

- *The Regenerative Community* builds community, makes new connections between people, and opens the way to explore meaning in life.
- *Resident-Directed Care* aims to restore control to the resident.
- *Individualized Care* helps residents return to familiar and comfortable routines.
- *The Eden Alternative* restores social and biological diversity and brings richness, spontaneity, and greater normalcy to daily life. (Fagan, Burger, and Williams, 1997, p. 35; see Thomas, 1996)

These pioneers bring great hope to connecting long-term care and spiritual well-being to nursing home life. (See also Binstock, Cluff, and Von Mering, 1996, and Bogenschneider and Olson, 1999.)

CONCLUSION

Spirituality and aging recommendations through four White House Conferences on Aging admonished faith congregations to reach out to members, to monitor institutions, and to offer services for older adults. The recommendations further asked the government to reach out to religious partners and to recognize the spiritual value of older persons in its public policy decisions.

During the same thirty-five years, public policy, often disconnected and ill-thought-out, was building a system of long-term care (primarily nursing home care) that neither in its design nor in reality provides for structures or services that recognize the value, worth, and spiritual well-being of older persons.

It is a hopeful sign that the spiritual issues that lead to the emptiness and lack of meaning of nursing home residents are being addressed by some practitioners, even though those issues are not being addressed in public policy funding, law, or regulations.

There clearly is a disconnection between spiritual well-being and long- term care public policy. The challenge therefore remains for both religious congregations and government to make changes in long-term care policy so that the spiritual needs of elders for relationships with God, community, and their environment will be met, no matter the setting.

REFERENCES

Binstock, Robert H., Leighton E. Cluff, and Otto Von Mering (Eds.) (1996). *The future of long-term care—Social and policy issues.* Baltimore MD: The Johns Hopkins University Press.

Bogenschneider, Karen and Jonathan Olson (Eds.) (1999). *Long-term care: State policy perspectives.* Madison, WI: Cooperative Extension Publications.

Coleman, Barbara (1996). *New directions for state long-term care systems—Volume I: Overview* (#9602). Washington, DC: AARP, Public Policy Institute.

Ellor, James W. (1997). Spiritual well-being defined. *Aging & Spirituality* 9(1):1.

Fagan, Rose Marie, Sarah Greene Burger, and Carter Catlett Williams (1997). *Meeting of pioneers in nursing home culture change.* Rochester, NY: LIFESPAN of Greater Rochester.

Families USA Foundation (1993). *The heavy burden of home care.* Washington, DC.

Friedman, Dayle (1995). The spiritual challenges of nursing home care. In Kimble, Melvin A., Susan H. McFadden, James W. Ellor, and James J. Seeber (Eds.), *Aging, spirituality, and religion* (pp. 362-373). Minneapolis, MN: Augsburg Fortress.

Holstein, Martha and Thomas Cole (1996). The evolution of long-term care in America. In Binstock, Robert H., Leighton E. Cluff, and Otto Von Mering (Eds.), *The future of long-term social and policy issues* (pp. 19-47). Baltimore, MD: The Johns Hopkins University Press.

Inventory of Recommendations for the 1971 White House Conference on Aging, No. 42 (1971). 1961 White House Conference on Aging. Washington, DC, AARP National Retired Teachers Association.

Kane, Rosalie (1998). Getting serious about quality of life in nursing homes. *Critical issues in aging* (No. 2, pp. 51-52). San Francisco: American Society on Aging.

Moberg, David O. (1971). *Spiritual well-being: Background and issues.* Washington, DC, 1971 White House Conference on Aging. U.S. Government Printing Office.

National Interfaith Coalition on Aging (NICA) (1975). *Spiritual well-being.* Athens, GA: NICA.

Polivka, Larry (1998). Long-term care advocacy. *Aging Research & Policy Report* (No. 8). Tampa, FL: Florida Policy Exchange Center on Aging.

Stone, Robyn (1999). Long-term care: Coming of age in the 21st century. In Bogenschneider, Karen and Jonathan Olson (Eds.), *Long-term care: State policy perspectives* (pp. 1-11). Madison, WI: Cooperative Extension Publications.

Thomas, William H. (1996). *Life worth living: How someone you love can still enjoy life in a nursing home—The Eden Alternative in action.* Acton, MA: VanderWyk and Burnham.

Vladeck, Bruce (1998). The future of home- and community-based long-term care. *Aging Research & Policy Report* (No. 8). Tampa, FL: Florida Policy Exchange Center on Aging.

White House Conference on Aging (1961). Reprinted in *Inventory of recommendations for the 1971 WHCA by AARP National Retired Teachers Association.* Washington, DC: U.S. Government Printing Office.

_____(1971a). *Spiritual well-being.* Washington, DC: U.S. Government Printing Office.

_____(1971b). *Toward a national policy on aging/Final report, II.* Washington, DC: U.S. Government Printing Office.

_____(1981). *Committee's recommendations from the White House Conference on Aging, November 30-December 3, 1981.* Washington, DC: U.S. Government Printing Office.

_____(1995a). *Official 1995 White House Conference on Aging—Adopted resolutions.* Washington, DC: U.S. Government Printing Office.

_____(1995b). *Official 1995 White House Conference on Aging—Final resolutions.* Washington, DC: U.S. Government Printing Office.

_____(1996, February). *Road to an aging policy for the 21st century—Final report.* Washington, DC: U.S. Government Printing Office.

Chapter 15

Guidelines for Research and Evaluation

David O. Moberg

Now that the importance of spirituality is generally recognized, one of the great needs is for research to clarify its impact and implications. "The interest and momentum in the study of aging, religion, and spirituality can be expected to continue to escalate. This will translate into research that asks new questions, probes for depth, and employs different methodologies. . . . Fortunately, a new climate of legitimacy for seeking answers to these questions awaits researchers willing to explore the interface between religion and aging" (Payne, 1995, p. 565).

Currently service organizations of all kinds are drawing up mission statements as a guide to action, a basis for evaluating the bottom-line financial and humanitarian outcomes of their work, and a step toward determining whether they are reaching their goals. Their assessments often require measuring tools and techniques to evaluate spirituality and other topics. Some excellent scales already are available (Hill and Hood, 1999; MacDonald et al., 1995; MacDonald, Friedman, and Kuentzel, 1999; MacDonald, Kuentzel, and Friedman, 1999), but many can lead to false conclusions, so it is very important to be keenly aware of criteria and methods for judging their strengths and weaknesses.

There are many ideologies, beliefs, and myths about the relationships between spirituality and other human concerns. We need to learn which among them are supported by evidence that is stronger than shallow opinions. Which types of spirituality are wholesomely related to physical and mental well-being? Which negatively? Which are consistent with the sacred scriptures and beliefs, respectively, of Judaism, Christianity, Islam, Buddhism, and Hinduism, and which are not? Are all religiously based spiritualities equivalent to each other so that it it does not matter what one's religion is, just so it is sincere? Or do some clash with and contradict others? Does spirituality have a genetic base, or is it entirely a learned phenomenon? What do the research findings imply for professional services that relate to reviving the human spirit, healing its ailments, and using its assets to improve personal and social life worldwide?

Obviously, questions like these call for research that draws upon the perspectives and expertise of numerous fields of investigation, including the humanities, biochemistry, and probably quantum physics, besides the social and behavioral sciences. Yet, as discussed in Chapter 1, basic philosophical assumptions and ideological commitments are foundation stones for each discipline and every theoretical and methodological orientation within it. These assumptions and ideologies should be called to attention whenever attempts are made to compare the findings of research projects, whether the studies are primarily scientific or applied. Only after extensive research on spirituality within particular frames of reference will it be possible to equitably compare and contrast the various definitions, methodologies, and professional applications connected with them in order to reach conclusions about spirituality that arc valid for all humanity (Moberg, 1997).

SPIRITUALITY MEASUREMENT
AND ASSESSMENT ISSUES

The following guidelines, principles, and precautions for studying and evaluating spirituality apply to doing research, assessing human services, and checking informally on the effectiveness of programs and activities intended to enhance spirituality. They provide important criteria for appraising the strengths and weaknesses of published or unpublished research done by others. They focus upon spirituality but cut across every type of pragmatic evaluation and scholarly research. While they emphasize methods that provide statistical data to test relationships among variables, they also apply to qualitative investigations outside the domain of statistics (see Reker, 1995).

These general guidelines apply to most, if not all, approaches to assessing the spirituality of elders, evaluating professional programs, and checking up on service delivery. Because much of the scientific research on spirituality has focused on spiritual well-being (SWB) and closely related concepts like spiritual maturity, SWB is used for examples of issues that arise in the measurement of religion and spirituality.

Identify and Control Your Personal Biases and Those of Your Profession

Biases tend to intrude into every stage of the research process, from the choice of topics believed worthy of investigation to final conclusions and reports. For example, explorations in mental health research have shown a general lack of interest in the subject of religion, misinterpretation of religious issues, low rates of theistic beliefs among mental health professions, high rates of apostasy from theistic family backgrounds, strong influence from psychoanalytic values, and failure to work together with the clergy to benefit clients who have a significant religious commitment (Larson, Sherrill, and Lyons, 1994). It is very easy to unconsciously give special attention to evidence that supports one's personal values and to overlook evidence that contradicts them but that others consider just as compelling. The ethic of honesty demands that we not ignore, distort, or rationalize away information that runs counter to our desires or expectations.

Develop Clear, Unambiguous Working Definitions

Developing working definitions is a crucial step in research and evaluation. The diversity of viewpoints about the nature of spirituality (Chapter 1) is of concern here. It is very complicated, seemingly ineffable, ephemeral, inscrutable, invisible, diffusely interwoven into all human beings and their behavior, and so transcendent that we cannot observe it directly with the human senses upon which all sciences rely. Arguably, it is the essence of our humanity, so we cannot step away from it to observe it from a distance. But similar limitations are true of many subjects of research (e.g., anomie, happiness, love, intelligence, loneliness, mental conditions, motivation, and prejudice) that can be studied only indirectly. That it is difficult to define SWB does not in itself make it unresearchable.

Spirituality overlaps so much with religion that many of its manifestations are also those of religiousness. But the two are not incompatible opposites, as if one who is spiritual cannot be religious, nor is either concept entirely subsumed in the other. Most people of faith combine expressions of religion with their spirituality. They attend religious services and support a religious group that nurtures their spiritual lives, on the one hand, and they engage in private spiritual practices that usually strengthen the loyalty to their religion, on the other.

The conceptual boundaries of both spirituality and religion often have been too narrow or too broad. Either extreme can impede good research. Many tools designed to measure either spirituality or religiousness actually measure aspects of both. Both domains may relate to the outcomes that a given research project investigates, so it often is more important to pay attention to specific components of the measures than to the spirituality or religiosity label assigned to it in a given study.

Since spirituality is defined in dozens, perhaps even hundreds, of ways, does your working definition imply that it is only religion? A purely subjective combination of feeling states? A specified set of activities? A relationship with God? Social relationships in a religious environment? A sensing of "The Holy" or sacred? To define it so that it fits every conceivable perspective is impossible. Instead, delimit it in the form of an operational definition that meets the needs of your investigation. You might, for example, say, "For the purposes of this study, we will assume that high levels of SWB consist of [name the specific actions by people; or attitudes expressed in interviews; or other observable phenomena, or combinations of answers to questionnaire items] and that low levels of SWB consist of [their counterparts]."

Measure Spirituality by Using Empirically Observable Indicators

These indicators reflect spirituality's presence or absence. To evaluate honestly the outcomes of any program intended to enhance spirituality or to reveal its relationship to other variables, it is necessary to devise observational techniques and instruments that we expect will identify and measure it. These usually take the form of questions for qualitative interviews, quantitative indexes or scales to summarize data from questionnaires or other sources, or findings from observational techniques of an academic discipline or profession. But still realize that it is possible to miss spirituality's essence, to choose indicators that do not truly reflect it, and to omit others that are more important.

Remember that SWB Is Multidimensional

Neither spirituality nor religiosity can be adequately evaluated by any single-item measure. (No single component of religion, such as measuring church attendance by the percentage of church members at Sunday worship services, evaluates religion as a whole.) These are complex concepts, so as many aspects as feasible should be included in the operational definition.

Just as there are many components of physical or mental health, there are many potential indicators of SWB (probably thousands). Every attempt to measure it uses only a tiny sample of them. Those selected are based upon previous knowledge, assumptions, theories, religious ideologies, and other value-based presuppositions that usually are unspoken. (Note that the word *evaluation* has *value* as its center.) If there are a thousand potential items and we use only ten, our sample of definitional variables may be considerably different from the sample of ten chosen by another researcher.

Comparisons of the findings of numerous studies that use diverse assessment tools, alongside studies to compare and improve those tools, are needed. Their findings may confirm each other, or they may expose clashes and disagreements that call for further investigation, plus components of spirituality that were overlooked or neglected.

The same complexity applies to every operational definition of a cause, effect, or correlate of SWB investigated. In the social and behavioral sciences, these are typically measured by scales or indexes, each of which combines several variables (most often answers to questions) to provide a single score. In the health sciences, for example, the outcomes observed typically are death or recovery from illness, length of hospital stay, the time lapse between services offered and recovery, and the need for and reactions to therapy or medications.

Sample All Indicators Carefully

Seldom do resources permit studying every person or project that is a part of whatever we investigate, so a few are chosen to represent the entire category. Good research tests whether those included are genuinely representative. Poor research, even by sincere persons or agencies, is dishonest if it claims that thousands of returns, as from a questionnaire sent to people known in advance to be on one side of a politically charged issue, prove that a majority of the nation is represented by their opinions. Representativeness is more important then large numbers.

Sampling also applies to choosing the components for measuring spirituality, as well as to choosing measures of the outcomes of spirituality and any other variables we wish to relate to it. Why, how, and with what assumptions and precedents do we choose those that are the focus of our attention? Are they the best measures? Do they genuinely represent all the measures that could have been selected?

Aim for a High Epistemic Correlation

Epistemic issues are present whenever two variables are related to each other. (The word is from epistemology, the branch of philosophy that deals with the origins, nature, methods, and limits of human knowledge, so *epistemic* pertains to knowledge and conditions for attaining it.) For example, if we speculate that the higher the average level of SWB of a group, the greater on average is its happiness, we test that hypothesis by discovering whether our measures of SWB and of happiness are correlated with each other. However, we cannot measure SWB and happiness directly, but only by observable indicators assumed to provide adequate measures. The relationship between each phenomenon (the actual or real A > B) and the measure of each (scale A > scale B) is the epistemic relationship. Good research requires a high epistemic correlation between spirituality-as-measured and genuine-or-true-spirituality. Seldom if ever are there unquestionably perfect epistemic correlations in any human sciences research (not only in studies of religion and spirituality).

Avoid the Fallacy of Reification

The mere existence of a word does not establish the reality it alleges (e.g., phlogiston is nonexistent). Nor does the ontological reality of spirituality consist only of whatever is included in an operational definition of SWB. The operations and criteria used in research should reflect the larger phenomenon of true SWB sufficiently to serve our research purposes, even as we simultaneously acknowledge that its reality may extend far beyond whatever we measure.

Avoid Reductionism

Do not treat empirical measures as if they represent the complete underlying reality of spirituality. Resist the ever-present temptation to assume that the actual phenomenon of spirituality is *nothing but* its measure, or that it consists of *only* its social, economic, physical, emotional, psychic, genetic, familial, ethical, moral, behavioral, or other measurable effects or accompaniments.

Be Honest in Your Analysis of Research Findings

Control your biases and be fair to those whose perspectives and values about spirituality differ from your own. For example, "fishing" in statistical data sets by trying one formula after another until one of them reveals statistically significant results may be shrewd, but if it violates assumptions beneath the statistical procedures chosen, it can foist deceit upon your analysis of the data.

Pay Attention to Emic and Etic Perspectives

The emic interpretations on what constitutes spiritual wellness and illness, those of a group under investigation, may differ from the etic views of outsiders, including researchers and scholars who try to be objective but have their own criteria for SWB and research goals (see Headland, Pike, and Harris, 1990). Significant ethical questions can be raised about the propriety and rightness of imposing outsiders' values upon a group, and that most of all if it leads to warfare, forced "conversions," colonization, or other compulsion. The imposition of various untested or inadequately verified (etic) assumptions with respect to African-American religion have fostered simplistic stereotypical views that impede the recognition that more complex models of black religiosity are necessary (Chatters and Taylor, 1994).

Avoid the "Ecological Fallacy"

This is the assumption that if a population as a whole, or a type of program or agency in general, has certain features, then every unit (person, program, agency) that is a part of it shares all of the same features (Moberg, 1983). We do not make this mistake by assuming that the average age of a group of people is the age of each member, but we are tempted to do so with respect to qualitative characteristics. For example, people who are deeply spiritual usually are also very religious, but that does not necessarily mean that every strongly religious person is deeply spiritual. We also must take care not to make this mistake when we generalize from the results of but one or a few studies. (Findings about the spirituality of Catholic Mexican-American farm laborers do not necessarily apply to Irish Catholic policemen, and vice versa.)

Test the Validity of Your Measurements

Do they genuinely measure spirituality? Researchers use three main methods to check the validity of a research instrument (i.e., to discover whether it actually measures the concept that it allegedly measures): face validity, criterion validity, and construct validity.

Face Validity (Sometimes Called Content Validity)

Face validity or content validity is simply the opinion of an investigator that a SWB scale really does measure SWB and, ideally, that it has a sufficient sample of components or indicators of SWB to do so adequately. The dependability of this twofold judgment hinges upon the investigator's definition of SWB, grasp of present knowledge of the subject, ideological and theoretical position with reference to SWB, and choice of indicators. (Are they truly germane to SWB as a whole and adequate to cover its main components?)

Problems emerge when there is disagreement about the definition or when the SWB scale seems to measure a different concept (e.g., religious ritualism, commitment to a particular faith, general life satisfaction, emotional feeling tones, self-actualization, caring behavior, serenity, etc.) instead of spirituality. These could be indicators, correlates, or reflectors of SWB, but that does not make them its essence.

Criterion Validity

Criterion validity involves any of at least five techniques:

1. *Pragmatic validity.* Does the SWB scale distinguish between subgroups of people who differ from each other with respect to SWB? For example, do persons or groups otherwise known to have high levels of SWB or to rate higher on components such as serenity score higher on the scale being tested than those who have low levels?

2. *Expert opinion.* Ask several SWB experts independently to evaluate each component (such as each survey question) as to whether and how responses to it distinguish between persons with high and low SWB.

3. *Concurrent validity.* Compare the scores of many persons on your new scale with their scores on a previously validated SWB instrument. If results are similar (correlated positively), the new scale has criterion validity.

But if there already is a scale, why develop a new one? Because the old scale may not sample enough components of SWB or may be cumbersome to use, too long, difficult for people with less than college education, filled with outmoded language ("he" and "man" for "all humans," Negro or black instead of African American, "thee" and "thy" religious phraseology, etc.), or use language that fits one religion better than another (homily versus sermon; priest versus minister, pastor, or rabbi; liturgy versus "order of worship"; parish or stake versus congregation, etc.).

4. *Predictive validity.* One could use SWB scores to predict what will happen in the future, then wait for future events; the scale is valid if its predictions come true. This is not easy with regard to spirituality. (In the Christian frame of reference the ultimate test is God's final judgment in the afterlife!) In societies that imprison, torture, or kill converts to Christian faith, one could predict that those with the highest SWB scores will be the most likely to remain true to their faith. In the United States they may be the most likely to support activities requiring costly commitment.

5. *Postdictive [retrospective] validity.* In some types of research it might be possible to compare current SWB scores with past approximations based upon the same persons' records, reports, memories, or

recollected beliefs and feeling states five, ten, or more years earlier. If the after/previous agreement is generally high, if there are good explanations of any discrepancies, and especially if one accepts continuity theory, validity of the indicators used is supported.

Construct Validity

Construct validity is the strongest, but also most complicated, test. It requires two or more "constructs" (measures, indexes, or scales) to measure SWB in order to test a particular hypothesis. For example, we could hypothesize that people in their seventies who have high levels of SWB (the *independent* or *causal variable*) will have fewer incidents of cardiopulmonary disease during the next twelve months (the *dependent* or *effect variable*) than otherwise similar persons with low levels of SWB. Assuming the diagnoses of the diseases are valid and reliable and that *intervening variables* such as smoking, diet, and exercise are controlled, we could test the hypothesis first with an already validated SWB Scale, then independently with the new SWB Scale. If findings from both tests are the same, the new scale has construct validity.

Thus one could apply the widely used Ellison-Paloutzian SWB Scale (see both Ledbetter et al., 1991 references) to test the validity of a new SWB scale that probes additional or alternative components, such as the interpersonal aspects of their horizonal dimension. Similarly, one could compare the same persons' scores on a Spiritual Maturity Scale with those on the SWB scale, assuming that high spiritual maturity occurs only among persons with high SWB (see Chapter 4, this volume; Genia, 1991; Hall et al., 1998).

Sometimes reference is made to *external validity,* validity tests in situations outside of the original study that generated a scale. It overlaps with criterion validity, reliability, and issues of sampling various populations. Most validity tests are *internal,* i.e., applied only within a given study.

Determine Whether Your Measurements Are Reliable

Even if a scale validly measures its intended concept, are its measurements accurate? Does it always give the same results when measuring the same thing? (For example, if your bathroom scale says you weigh 140 pounds but a minute later without ingesting or eliminating it reads 130, then in half an hour your physician's scale reports 160, your scale is not reliable.) The unreliability of a SWB scale based on a questionnaire may result from such problems as ambiguous answer categories (am I "average," "somewhat above average," or "high" on a question?), different interpretations of the wording of questions, or relationships of questions to one another that make savvy respondents avoid being "stung" by "trick questions" to test whether they are lying (perhaps reflecting their reliability instead of the instrument's).

There are four main ways to test reliability:

1. *Parallel (or multiple or alternate) forms* administered simultaneously. If they produce the same scores, the instrument is considered reliable.
2. *Repeated applications,* such as a week or month apart, of the same scale given to the same persons. A weakness is that different results may reflect actual changes, as in attitudes toward publicized news events related to spirituality. Another is reactivity; the first experience with the scale or its pleasant or distressing nature biases answers the second time. Sometimes the Hawthorne effect occurs—persons who know they are being studied may change their behavior during observation or testing. Questions in the scale may stimulate thinking about a topic not previously considered, so respondents may (a) modify their opinions, (b) answer the way they surmise the researcher or sponsor desires, or (c) state an opinion when they really have none.
3. For the *split-half method* the initial scale may have twice as many items as eventually desired or consist of Forms A and B. If the score on one half is the same as that on the other half (often split by alternate numbered items), the scale is reliable. But are the two halves actually equivalent? Might some items measure SWB status at the moment and others spiritual growth (progress) or maturity (attainment)? Thus this method needs the support of criterion validity.
4. *Statistical techniques* usually evaluate individual items in relationship to the total score on a scale. If an item scores high on persons whose overall score is low or on both high and low scoring persons, it can be rejected or rescored, modified, and retested on the next round of research.

Avoid Distorting Observations of Incidents and Events Related to Spirituality

Check on whether personal values or those of your culture or groups you are affiliated with distort your sensory observations, especially with reference to such matters as biases and the emic and etic perspectives discussed earlier. (This could result from commitment to a particular gerontological theory, religious group, ideology, therapeutic school, or other professional beliefs.) Ideally, we should try to see "all sides" of everything we investigate, not only the side that is personally most comfortable. Good research methods try honestly to see things as they really are, not only as we wish, hope, or expect them to be.

Report Your Research Findings Objectively and Fairly

Do not slant them by emotionally toned words and phrases that are unfair to those with whom you disagree. Openly identify and humbly share the boundaries, weaknesses, and limitations of your work.

CONCLUSIONS

We have seen that many research techniques and methods are as applicable to the study of spirituality as they are to other nonmaterial subjects. While spirituality and religiousness overlap so much that the two concepts may always be entangled with each other, various components of each can be separated, and each can be related to other research variables (Larson, Sherrill, and Lyons, 1994). The scholarly methods of investigation can be applied or adapted for administrative evaluations and assessments (see Sinnott et al., 1983), not used only in gerontological research.

Good research methods for investigating spirituality are grounded in a solid understanding of the assumptions and postulates upon which each methodology rests. They recognize alternative theoretical and theological views on spirituality. They are fully consistent with the Ten Commandments (Drees, 1998) and can be interpreted as applications of them. When they probe therapeutic techniques, they similarly reflect the ideological values that are the fountainhead of each approach. Scientific studies of spirituality support the virtues of truthfulness, honesty, and integrity and help us to improve people's lives.

REFERENCES

Chatters, Linda M. and Robert Joseph Taylor (1994). Religious involvement among older African-Americans. In Levin, Jeffrey S. (Ed.), *Religion in aging and health* (pp. 196-230). Thousand Oaks, CA: Sage Publications.

Drees, Willem B. (1998). Ten commandments for quality in science and spirituality. *Science & Spirit* 9(4):2-4.

Genia, Vicky (1991). The spiritual experience index: A measure of spiritual maturity. *Journal of Religion and Health* 30(4):337-347.

Hall, Todd W., Beth Fletcher Brokaw, Keith J. Edwards, and Patricia L. Pike (1998). An empirical exploration of psychoanalysis and religion: Spiritual maturity and object relations development. *Journal for the Scientific Study of Religion* 37(2):303-312.

Headland, Thomas N., Kenneth L. Pike, and Marvin Harris (Eds.) (1990). *Emics and etics: The insider/outsider debate* (Frontiers of Anthropology, Volume 7). Newbury Park, CA: Sage Publications.

Hill, Peter C. And Ralph W. Hood Jr. (Eds) (1999). *Measures of religiosity*. Birmingham, AL: Religion Education Press.

Larson, David B., Kimberly A. Sherrill, and John S. Lyons (1994). Neglect and misuse of the R word. In Levin, Jeffrey S. (Ed.), *Religion in aging and health* (pp. 178-195). Thousand Oaks, CA: Sage Publications.

Ledbetter, M. F., L. A. Smith, J. D. Fischer, and W. L. Vosler-Hunter (1991). An evaluation of the construct validity of the Spiritual Well-Being Scale: A factor-analytic approach. *Journal of Psychology and Theology* 19(1):94-103.

Ledbetter, M. F., L. A. Smith, W. L. Vosler-Hunter, and J. D. Fischer (1991). An evaluation of the research and clinical usefulness of the Spiritual Well-Being Scale. *Journal of Psychology and Theology* 19(1):49-55.

MacDonald, Douglas A., H. L. Friedman, and J. G. Kuentzel (1999). A survey of measures of spiritual and transpersonal constructs: Part one—Research update. *Journal of Transpersonal Psychology* 31(2):137-154.

MacDonald, Douglas A., J. G. Kuentzel, and H. L. Friedman (1999). A survey of measures of spiritual and transpersonal constructs: Part two—Additional instruments. *Journal of Transpersonal Psychology* 31(2):155-177.

MacDonald, Douglas A., L. LeClair, C. J. Holland, A. Alter, and H. L. Friedman (1995). A survey of measures of spiritual and transpersonal constructs. *Journal of Transpersonal Psychology* 27(2):171-235.

Moberg, David O. (1983). The ecological fallacy: Concerns for program planners. *Generations* 8(1):12-14.

Moberg, David O. (1997). "Tensions between universalism and particularism in research on spiritual well-being." Paper presented at the joint annual meeting of the Illinois and Wisconsin Sociological Associations, Rockford, IL, October 31.

Payne, Barbara Pittard (1995). The interdisciplinary study of gerontology. In Kimble, Melvin A., Susan H. McFadden, James W. Ellor, and James J. Seeber (Eds.), *Aging, spirituality, and religion* (pp. 558-567). Minneapolis, MN: Fortress Press.

Reker, Gary T. (1995). Quantitative and qualitative methods. In Kimble, Melvin A., Susan H. McFadden, James W. Ellor, and James J. Seeber (Eds.), *Aging, spirituality, and religion* (pp. 568-588). Minneapolis, MN: Fortress Press.

Sinnott, Jan D., Charles S. Harris, Marilyn R. Block, Stephen Collesano, and Solomon G. Jacobson (1983). *Applied research in aging: A guide to methods and resources.* Boston: Little, Brown and Co.

Chapter 16

Continuing Challenges

David O. Moberg

The channels for deepening and applying our understanding of spirituality are rapidly increasing. Every year, thousands of books and articles related to it are pouring off the popular and scholarly presses, and the Internet has an abundance of related listings. Religious organizations of all stripes are giving it increasing attention. Yet Peterson (1997) believes that, although this interest reflects a secularized society in which people are searching for a spiritual anchor, the frequency with which the word spirituality is used is more likely an evidence of pathology than of health.

THE BABEL OF SPIRITUALITY CONCEPTS

There still is such a wide variety of explicit and implicit definitions of spirituality and related words that one seldom can be sure that two similar-sounding accounts actually deal with the same subject. Some confuse spirituality with concepts of physical and mental health, while others focus upon internalized feelings, even to the exclusion of behavior. Institutionalized religion rather than personal spirituality grabs the attention of many. Some who use the word are in the spirit of biblical Judaism or Christianity, but others reflect ancient contrasting or clashing spirits of earth worship, astrological religions, or fertility goddesses.

Instead of casually using the rubric of spirituality, we therefore must examine such details as the philosophical and theological assumptions in the essays and speeches that use the word, in operational definitions applied in its research, in professional theories of the human services that recognize its value, and in beliefs and commitments that lurk beneath each spiritual exercise and spirituality workshop.

A few words quoted from the Qur'an or from the records of Jesus in the Christian gospels do not by themselves make a presentation genuinely Muslim or Christian. Neither does a label for the type of spiritual therapy used by a counselor necessarily make his or her therapeutic interventions equivalent to those of other therapists who use the same label. Divergent spiritual commitments, not only different situational perspectives for viewing the issues, pervade the public square and help to color much current controversy over such issues as abortion, euthanasia, homosexuality, sex education, and physician-assisted suicide.

SPIRITUAL DIVERSITY

The population of the United States is increasingly "a tapestry woven of many different strands" (Lipson, Dibble, and Minarik, 1996, p. iv). Its people, from all parts of the world, have vast cultural differences, not the least of which are variations in religious and spiritual traditions. Even though theological and moral values derived from European culture and the Christian religion are still dominant, there are wide variations within them and even greater contrasts with traditions from Asian, African, and Oceanic societies.

Cross-cultural misunderstandings easily emerge from these differences. The manual by Lipson, Dibble, and Minarik (1996) is an outstanding reference work for anyone working with diverse types of people. It describes the cultural identity, communication patterns, activities of daily living, food practices, symptom management in illness, birth and death rituals, family relationships, illness beliefs, health practices, and spiritual/religious orientations of two dozen cultural groups plus ten spiritual and religious groups. It reminds readers that the actions, words, symbols, rituals, and therapeutic interventions that help people of one culture group sometimes annoy or even harm persons from others.

In Islam, both health and illness are believed to come from God, so the art of healing is closely linked to worship. "The body itself is seen as a mere receptacle for the spirit, which alone constitutes the immortal part of human existence. . . . Healing through supplications, prayers, and fasting is a well-established tradition in Islam" (Iqbal, 1998, pp. 34-35). Devout Muslims gain psychological and social benefits from their submission or surrender of the whole self to God, adherence to the rituals of ablution, prayer, fasting, alms giving, one or more pilgrimages to Mecca, and conformity to rules for daily living (Azayem and Hedayat-Diba, 1994).

Religiously committed Buddhists, Hindus, Jews, Native Americans, Sikhs, Christian Scientists, Jehovah's Witnesses, Mormons, and members of many Christian denominations have distinctive theological doctrines and behavioral customs that influence their attitudes, beliefs, and behavior related to spirituality, as well as toward therapeutic interventions in the caring professions. Sensitivity to their faith and civil liberties should dominate all research and professional work with them.

ASSESSING AND MEASURING SPIRITUALITY

Although we have covered a wide range of both scholarly investigations and applied programs in the field of spirituality and aging, the subject is so vast that we have only scratched the surface. Religion and spirituality are considered important by such a large proportion of people that one would expect religious and spiritual indicators to be included among the dimensions or components measured in quality of life instruments (Moberg, 1979). Such, however, still is not the case. Spirituality is almost always ignored, even in multidimensional assessments (see Fletcher, Dickinson, and Philp, 1992). One reason may be its complexity. Assessment tools and measurement techniques easily pick up one or a few of its facets while ignoring dozens of others that are equally or more important, as dicussed in Chapters 4 and 15.

All of the research to date needs to be replicated, extended, and refined. Countless specialized topics deserve further attention. For example, the work on prayer in relationship to well-being (Chapter 4) is in its infancy. The various kinds of prayer (petition, intercession, confession, praise, thanksgiving, etc.), as well as its styles (individual, group, liturgical, meditative, musical, tongues, sacrifices, etc.) and to whom it is addressed (God, Allah, Christ, self, Gaia, etc.), are but a few of its dimensions that could be studied in relationship to health, serenity, social justice, or other desired outcomes. Similarly, the effects of various therapeutic theories and techniques related to spirituality can be tested, and research can explore topics such as love, friendship, forgiveness, and effects of the various theodicies and meanings attached to death (see Moberg, 1981) that presumably influence and are influenced by spirituality.

Even the best methodologies for spirituality research are not perfect. Perhaps none ever will be. This is not a valid excuse to give up research, however. As in every area of investigation, we must use the best tools available, always recognizing that all are limited. Their findings are always tentative and provisional, needing confirmation by replications on a wide range of people in a variety of social and cultural contexts.

Most research to date has centered around generalized forms of "American spirituality." It now needs to be sharpened in several directions. One is to conduct more studies in Christian subgroups like evangelicals and fundamentalists to determine whether (as some research already suggests) people with those orientations have different levels of well-being and life satisfaction from those whose Christian views are anchored in theological liberalism, traditional Roman Catholicism, or Eastern Orthodoxy. Another is to compare the manner and extent to which atheistic, New Age, Hindu, Buddhist, Muslim, Orthodox and Reform Jewish, Catholic, Protestant, and other religious and philosophical spiritual commitments relate to specific measures of human well-being. Only after these and other "particularistic" studies have been made can we determine empirically whether there is a "universalistic" relationship (applying generally to all humanity) between spirituality and other indicators of satisfaction, happiness, health, and well-being (Moberg, in press).

SPIRITUALITY IN HEALTH CARE

The importance of spirituality is increasingly recognized in health care (Chapters 7 and 8). Spiritual care is a necessary role of nurses whenever their concern includes the whole person (Shelly and Fish, 1988; Carson, 1989). A major concern of most hospice programs is the spiritual journey of their patients. The spirituality of physicians and other caregivers is now known to have an impact on patient care (Warde, 1999; Sulmasy, 1999).

Remarkable progress has been made in research on the epidemiology of religion. Nearly 80 percent of Americans believe in the power of God or of prayer to improve the course of illness. As of 1991, 70 percent of physicians reported religious inquiries for counseling on terminal illness, yet only 10 percent of them ever asked about their patients' beliefs or practices. That situation is changing under the impact of medical education and conferences demonstrating the importance of religion and spirituality in patients' lives (Levin, Larson, and Puchalski, 1997).

The number of U.S. medical schools offering courses in spirituality and medicine increased from three in 1995 to over sixty in 1999 (Larson, 1999). Many medical schools are teaching physicians how to make a spiritual assessment of patients. One way this is structured is by the acronym FICA, standing for *Faith* and belief, *Importance* and influence of faith, *Community* ("Are you part of a spiritual or religious community? . . ."), and *Address in care* ("How would you like me, your health care provider, to address these issues in your health care?"). This form of listening and love supports and encourages patients, and it strengthens rapport with their physicians. Whenever advisable, it expedites referral to chaplains, clergy, or spiritual counselors. It makes physician-patient interaction a concern for the whole person, improves the therapy, and deepens relationships between them (Puchalski, 1999a, b).

Nearly all problems dealt with in medicine have a spiritual dimension. Physicians, like other clinicians and therapists, nevertheless encounter dilemmas when they incorporate spiritual perspectives into their practice (Gruber, 1995). Sometimes prayers with patients become a form of manipulation of or by them. Patients may irritate their providers by denying a diagnosis, refusing or not following treatment, or annoying false "emergency" interruptions. The "secret language of the unconscious" intrudes. "Impaired spirituality creates obstacles to healing. Almost always the suffering patient becomes invested in control or power issues, maintaining a brittle self-concept, or struggles about dependency" (Gruber, 1995, p. 136).

False spirituality is ego-based and can affect both the healer and the patient. It easily masquerades as true, using the same terminology and rituals. True spirituality involves a willing surrender of both the patient and healer to the demands of life, to service, to each other, and to the will of God. It does not guarantee a cure. It "is not defined by saying certain words, or by a spiritual appearance, eloquence, by a distinguished presentation on television, by financial success, or by the approval of religious authorities" (Gruber, 1995, p. 136). It forms a deep empathetic relationship with the patient that enables "the ability to step into the client's private world so completely that all desire to evaluate is lost" (p. 138).

SPIRITUALITY IN OTHER PROFESSIONS

Awareness of the hunger for eternity that seems implanted in the human heart finds expression in most, if not all, spiritual paths of traditional religions, even if some of their religious leaders seem to have lost sight of the focus on spirituality that was central to their founders' work.

Many chapters in this book provide examples of the assimilation of spiritual concepts and care that is occurring in all human service occupations. Exploring the spiritual concerns of clients is of great help in family therapy (Fischer, 1992). Much of the success of Prison Fellowship and other nongovernmental ministries to prisoners and exoffenders flows from their explicit attention to spirituality (see Smarto, 1993). The same is true of Alcoholics Anonymous and many other self-help programs for people with addictions.

The code of ethics of the National Association of Social Workers requires social workers to be culturally competent in several areas, including spirituality and religion, but incorporating them into college teaching is challenging (e.g., Staral, 1999). Deficiencies of vocabulary and conspiracies of silence about inner experience are common in professional work in the field of aging, but they can be overcome by questions to draw out spiritual reflections that provide a rich source of insight (Atchley, 1999).

The principles and techniques for serving spiritual needs in any of these professions can be adapted for use in the others. So, too, can many of their instruments and techniques for assessing the spirituality of clients. For example, Boyd's (1988) Comprehensive Religious/ Spiritual Assessment Tool has questions in three major categories. The first deals with a client's *religious and spiritual history,* asking questions about religious upbringing, life-sharing experiences, conversion/peak/mystical experiences, spiritual crises and emergencies, and current social environment. The second part probes *current beliefs and practices,* including questions about religious identity; commitment level; religious identifications/affiliations/involvements; codification of beliefs; rituals, images, and symbols; behavioral enactments, observances, and practices; God image and theodicies; and concepts of evil and the demonic. Finally, *spiritual maturity and development* has sections on development through the stages of life, effect of religious/spiritual identity on life style, meaning of life issues, and moral frame of reference. All topics are especially useful for in-depth interviews, which should be adapted to fit each specific client and situation.

The conceptual framework for assessing the spiritual functioning and fulfillment of older adults in long-term settings developed by Thibault, Ellor, and Netting (1991) has similar content. It asks closed-end questions about thirteen needs related to the exterior/institutional domain, six needs related to the interior life domain, and three in the domain of belief/knowledge.

Collaboration among the various human service professions is often deficient, so they sometimes are seen as competing with each other, especially in regard to spirituality and religion, instead of working together on behalf of clients they mutually serve. A review of eight major psychological journals from 1991 to 1994 found that only four (0.02 percent) of 2,468 quantitative studies considered clergy in their data (Weaver et al., 1997). This suggests that psychologists have ignored the effects of clergy involvement in mental health care, despite the significant role they often play. Yet Koenig and Weaver (1997) have demonstrated how psychiatric and clinical knowledge about specific kinds of mental health problems of older adults can help the clergy know how best to respond to their diverse needs.

Professional practice is sometimes hampered or distorted by competing values regarding social ethics and public policy (see Holstein and Mitzen, 1998). The "separation of church and state" often overpowers the "freedom of religion" constitutional provisions. Neutrality toward all religions gravitates toward their exclusion while allowing, sometimes even encouraging, the intrusion of antireligious practices in the public square. In spite of some attention in the White House Conferences on Aging (see Chapter 14), serious dialogue about the appropriate role of the public sector in financing and providing a spiritual component as a part of health and human services has been conspiciously absent (Kapp, 1999). Traditional linkages of spirituality with religion and of government with nongovernmental agencies tend to impede explicit attention to people's spiritual needs in all human service professions and agencies.

SPIRITUALITY IN EVERYDAY LIFE

Spirituality is not a realm separate from daily living, much less an orientation of life or activity that is for religious rituals and places alone. Separation of the sacred from the secular has long been a flaw of Western civilization. The Creator is above and beyond time, yet it is "in him we live and move and have our being," as St. Paul reminded the philosophers of Athens long ago (Acts 17:28, NIV).

"Test everything. Hold on to the good. Avoid every kind of evil" (1 Thessalonians 5:21-22, NIV) is just as good advice to us today as it was to people in Greece nineteen centuries ago. The "Ignatian spirituality" of "contemplation in action" and "finding God in all things" is not for Jesuits and Catholics alone, but for all who believe in God. It is a "hidden spring" that opens awareness to God's presence in ordinary life. It guides people to a healthy spirituality out of which they worship God by putting themselves at the service of others in the midst of the world in which God is always present (Hart, 1994; Smith and Merz, 2000). Such service includes accepting the immense challenges of "spiritual gerontology and geriatrics" for contemporary society, and all of its institutions, organizations, and professions.

Most models of personal spirituality that are popular today "were primarily developed in the desert, behind cloistered walls, in the priest's vestry or the pastor's study" (Banks, 1998, p. 11), but that is not where most people live. What needs greater emphasis now is not only a spirituality of contemplation, but one of active life, a *spirituality of the center* rather than of the periphery, one rooted in everyday realities, not only those of the secluded inner life. It vigorously embraces and celebrates all of life and *practices the presence of God* in every activity, situation, and circumstance. It is a spirituality that all (professionals included) can engage in with eyes wide open while we go about the practical duties of life, not a spirituality to practice only on retreats or when eyes are meditatively shut (Banks, 1998). It is the way to "pray without ceasing" (1 Thessalonians 5:17) in the midst of a busy world.

REFERENCES

Atchley, Robert C. (1999). Incorporating spirituality into professional work in aging. *Aging Today* 20(4):17.

Azayem, Gamal Abou El and Zari Hedayat-Diba (1994). The psychological aspects of Islam: Basic principles of Islam and their psychological corollary. *International Journal for the Psychology of Religion* 4(1):41-50.

Banks, Rob (1998). Toward an eyes wide-open spirituality. *Faith at Work* 111(3, Fall):11.

Boyd, Timothy A. (1988). Spiritually sensitive assessment tools for social work practice. In Hugen, Beryl (Ed.), *Christianity and social work* (pp. 239-255). Botsford, CT: North American Association of Christians in Social Work.

Carson, Verna Benner (1989). *Spiritual dimensions of nursing practice.* Philadelphia: W. B. Saunders Co.

Fischer, Kathleen R. (1992). Spirituality and the aging family: A systems perspective. *Journal of Religious Gerontology* 8(4):1-15.

Fletcher, Astrid E., Edward J. Dickinson, and Ian Philp (1992). Review: Audit measures: Quality of life instruments for everyday use with elderly patients. *Age and Aging* 21(2):142-150.

Gruber, Louis N. (1995). True and false spirituality: A framework for Christian behavioral medicine. *Journal of Psychology and Christianity* 14(2):133-140.

Hart, Thomas (1994). *Hidden spring: The spiritual dimension of therapy.* Mahwah, NJ: Paulist Press.

Holstein, Martha and Phyllis Mitzen (Guest editors) (1998). Ethics and aging: Bringing the issues home. *Generations* (special issue) 22(1):3-104.

Iqbal, Muzaffar (1998). Islamic medicine: The tradition of spiritual healing. *Science & Spirit* 9(4): 34-36.

Kapp, Marshall B. (1999). Aging and public policy: Does spirituality have a role in health and human service programs? In Ellor, James, Susan McFadden, and Stephen Sapp (Eds.), *Aging & spirituality: The first decade* (pp. 110-113). San Francisco: American Society on Aging.

Koenig, Harold G. and Andrew J. Weaver (1997). *Counseling troubled older adults: A handbook for pastors and religious caregivers.* Nashville, TN: Abingdon Press.

Larson, David B. (1999). Letter from the president of the National Institute for Healthcare Research to David O. Moberg, August 12.

Levin, Jeffrey S., David B. Larson, and Christina M. Puchalski (1997). Religion and spirituality in medicine: Research and education. *Journal of the American Medical Association* 278(9):792-793.

Lipson, Juliene G., Suzanne L. Dibble, and Pamela A. Minarik (1996). *Culture & nursing: A pocket guide.* San Francisco: University of California San Francisco Nursing Press.

Moberg, David O. (1979). The development of social indicators for quality of life research. *Sociological Analysis* 40(1):11-26.

Moberg, David O. (1981). Spiritual well-being of the dying. In Lesnoff-Caravaglia, Gari (Ed.), *Aging and the human condition* (pp. 139-155). New York: Human Sciences Press.

Moberg, David O. (In press). Assessing and measuring spirituality: Confronting dilemmas of universal and particular evaluative criteria. *Journal of Adult Development.*

NIV: *The Holy Bible,* New International Version (1984). Colorado Springs, CO: International Bible Society.

Peterson, Eugene H. (1997). *Subversive spirituality.* Grand Rapids, MI: Eerdmans.

Puchalski, Christina M. (1999a). A spiritual assessment: Listening to your patients. *Spirituality & Medicine Connection* 3(1, Spring):3.

Puchalski, Christina M. (1999b). Taking a spiritual history: FICA. *Spirituality & Medicine Connection* 3(1, Spring):1.

Shelly, Judith Allen and Sharon Fish. (1988). *Spiritual care: The nurse's role* (Third edition). Downers Grove, IL: InterVarsity Press.

Smarto, Don. (Ed.). (1993). *Setting the captives free! Relevant ideas in criminal justice and prison ministry.* Grand Rapids, MI: Baker Book company

Smith, Carol Ann, SHCJ and Eugene F. Merz, SJ (2000). *Moment by moment: A retreat in everyday life.* Norte Dame, IN: Ave Maria Press.

Staral, Janice M. (1999). Seeking religious and spiritual competence: The perceptions of BSW students at a private Catholic university. *Social Work and Christianity* 26(2):101-111.

Sulmasy, Daniel (1999). Face to face: Interview. *Spirituality & Medicine Connection* 3(2):6.

Thibault, Jane M., James W. Ellor, and F. Ellen Netting (1991). A conceptual framework for assessing the spiritual functioning and fulfillment of older adults in long-term care settings. *Journal of Religious Gerontology* 7(4):29-45.

Warde, Deirdre (1999). Research review: The role of spirituality for healthcare providers. *Spirituality & Medicine Connection* 3(2):4.

Weaver, Andre J., Judith A. Samford, Amy E. Kline, Lee Ann Lucas, David B. Larson, and Harold G. Koenig (1997). What do psychologists know about working with the clergy? An analysis of eight APA journals: 1991-1994. *Professional Psychology: Research and Practice* 28(5):471-474.

Recommended Readings

Each chapter of this book refers to many resources for further study and reading about spirituality and aging. The body of knowledge on the subject is steadily and rapidly multiplying. The following are particularly relevant for building a solid foundation of in-depth understanding of various aspects of the subject and for applying those "lessons" in personal or professional life.

Ellor, James, Susan McFadden, and Stephen Sapp (Eds.) (1999). *Aging and spirituality: The first decade.* San Francisco: American Society on Aging. Selected articles from the first ten years of the quarterly newsletter of ASA's Forum on Religion, Spirituality, and Aging.

Hood, Ralph, W. Jr. (Ed.) (1995). *Handbook of religious experience.* Birmingham, AL: Religious Education Press. Psychological studies of religious experience within the context of six major faith traditions.

Journal of Religious Gerontology (Binghamton, NY: The Haworth Press, quarterly). An interdisciplinary and interfaith journal devoted to religion and aging.

Kimble, Melvin A., Susan H. McFadden, James W. Ellor, and James J. Seeber (Eds.) (1995). *Aging, spirituality, and religion: A handbook.* Minneapolis, MN: Fortress Press. A massive and masterful collection with forty chapters by specialists from diverse disciplines and professions; strongly recommended for all professional and agency libraries.

Koenig, Harold G. (1994). *Aging and God: Spiritual pathways to mental health in midlife and later years.* Binghamton, NY: The Haworth Press. Historical, theoretical, empirical, and clinical perspectives on religion/spirituality and mental health.

Koenig, Harold G. (1995). *Research on religion and aging: An annotated bibliography.* Westport, CT: Greenwood Press. Abstracts of 291 articles and books published from 1980 to 1995 along with Koenig's evaluation of the research quality of most entries.

Koenig, Harold G. (1997). *Is religion good for your health? The effects of religion on physical and mental health.* Binghamton, NY: The Haworth Press. A concise survey of the research evidence.

Larson, David B. and Susan Larson (1998). *Forgotten factor in physical and mental health: What does research show?* Rockville, MD: National Institute for Healthcare Research. A summary of research on the impact of religion/spirituality on health.

Levin, Jeffrey S. (Ed.) (1994). *Religion in aging and health: Theoretical foundations and methodological frontiers.* Thousand Oaks, CA: Sage Publications. Eight in-depth studies reporting, interpreting, and evaluating research that interfaces aspects of religion with aging and health.

Lipson, Juliene G., Suzanne L. Dibble, and Pamela A. Minarik (Eds.) (1996). *Culture and nursing care.* San Francisco: UCSF Nursing Press, 1996. An excellent compendium of the cultural and religious/spiritual orientations, rituals, and practices of twenty-four ethnic groups and ten religious groups encountered in nursing practice that is useful in all clinical professions.

Richards, P. Scott and Allen E. Bergin (1997). *A spiritual strategy for counseling and psychotherapy.* Washington, DC: American Psychological Association. A thoroughly documented study of the need for a strategy to incorporate spirituality in counseling, its historical, theoretical, and philosophical foundations, processes and methods of spiritual interventions, assessments and research, and future directions.

Shelly, Judith Allen and Sharon Fish (1988). *Spiritual care: The nurse's role,* Third edition. Downers Grove, IL: InterVarsity Press. Principles and procedures for sensitively addressing spiritual needs of patients that can be applied in every human profession.

Thomas, L. Eugene and Susan A. Eisenhandler. (Eds.) (1994). *Aging and the religious dimension.* Westport, CT: Auburn House, 1994. Narrative and qualitative research, historical and literary studies, and theoretical perspectives on religion and spirituality.

Person Index

Subject Index